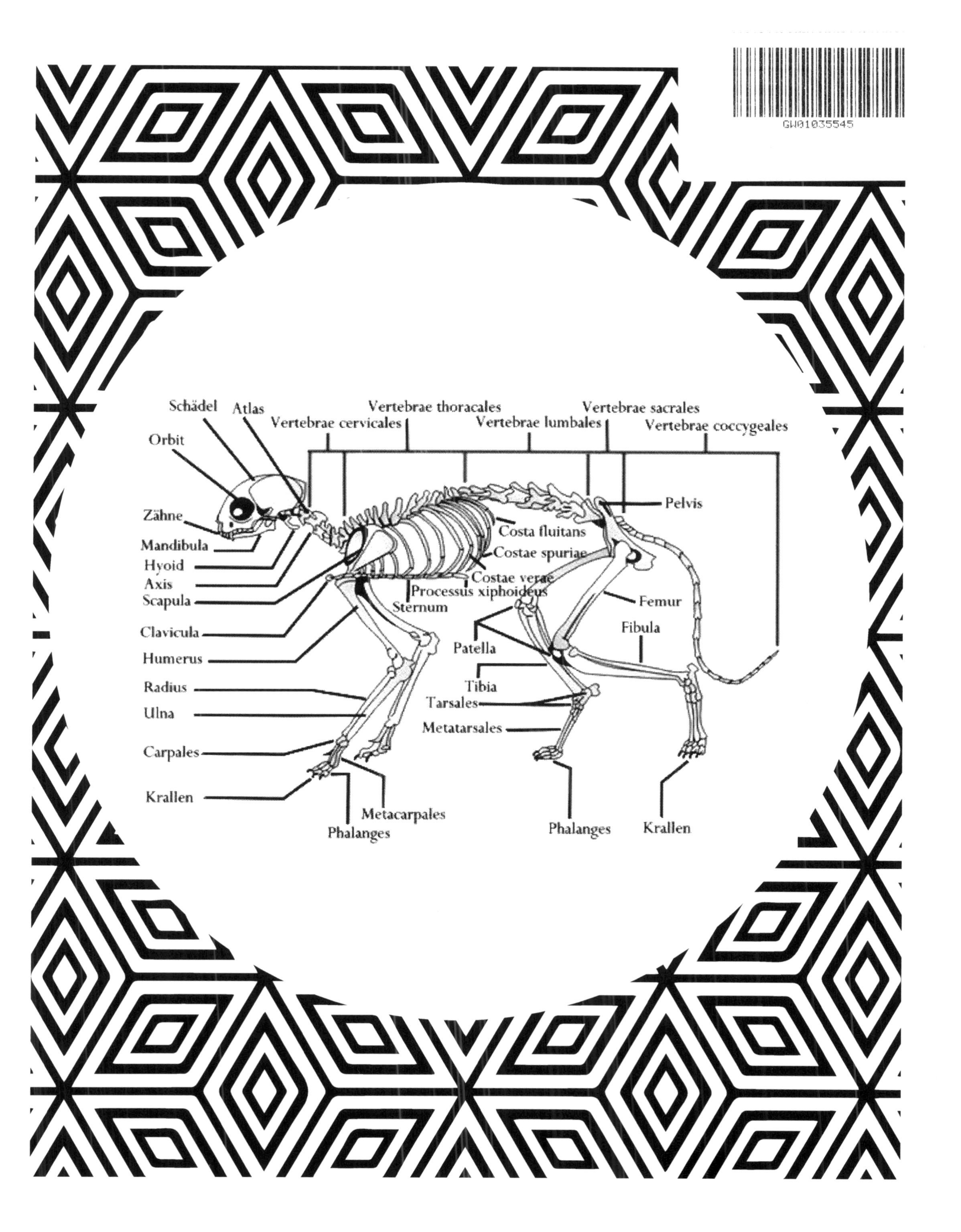

Schädel
Atlas
Vertebrae thoracales
Vertebrae sacrales
Vertebrae cervicales
Vertebrae lumbales
Vertebrae coccygeales
Orbit
Pelvis
Zähne
Costa fluitans
Mandibula
Costae spuriae
Hyoid
Costae verae
Axis
Processus xiphoideus
Scapula
Sternum
Femur
Clavicula
Fibula
Patella
Humerus
Tibia
Radius
Tarsales
Ulna
Metatarsales
Carpales
Krallen
Metacarpales
Phalanges
Phalanges
Krallen

This Book Belongs To

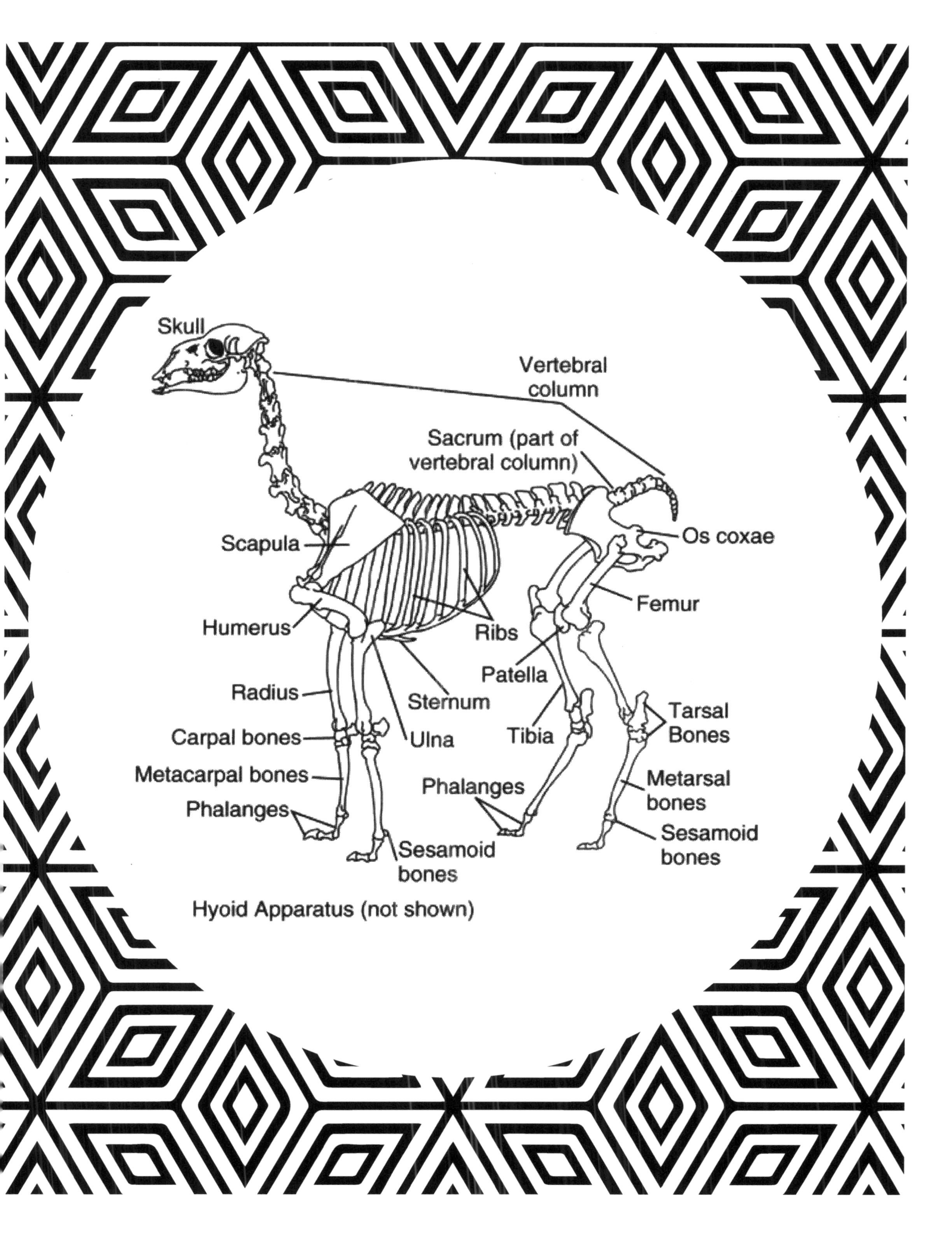
Skull
Vertebral column
Sacrum (part of vertebral column)
Os coxae
Scapula
Femur
Humerus
Ribs
Patella
Radius
Sternum
Tarsal Bones
Carpal bones
Ulna
Tibia
Metacarpal bones
Phalanges
Metarsal bones
Phalanges
Sesamoid bones
Sesamoid bones
Hyoid Apparatus (not shown)

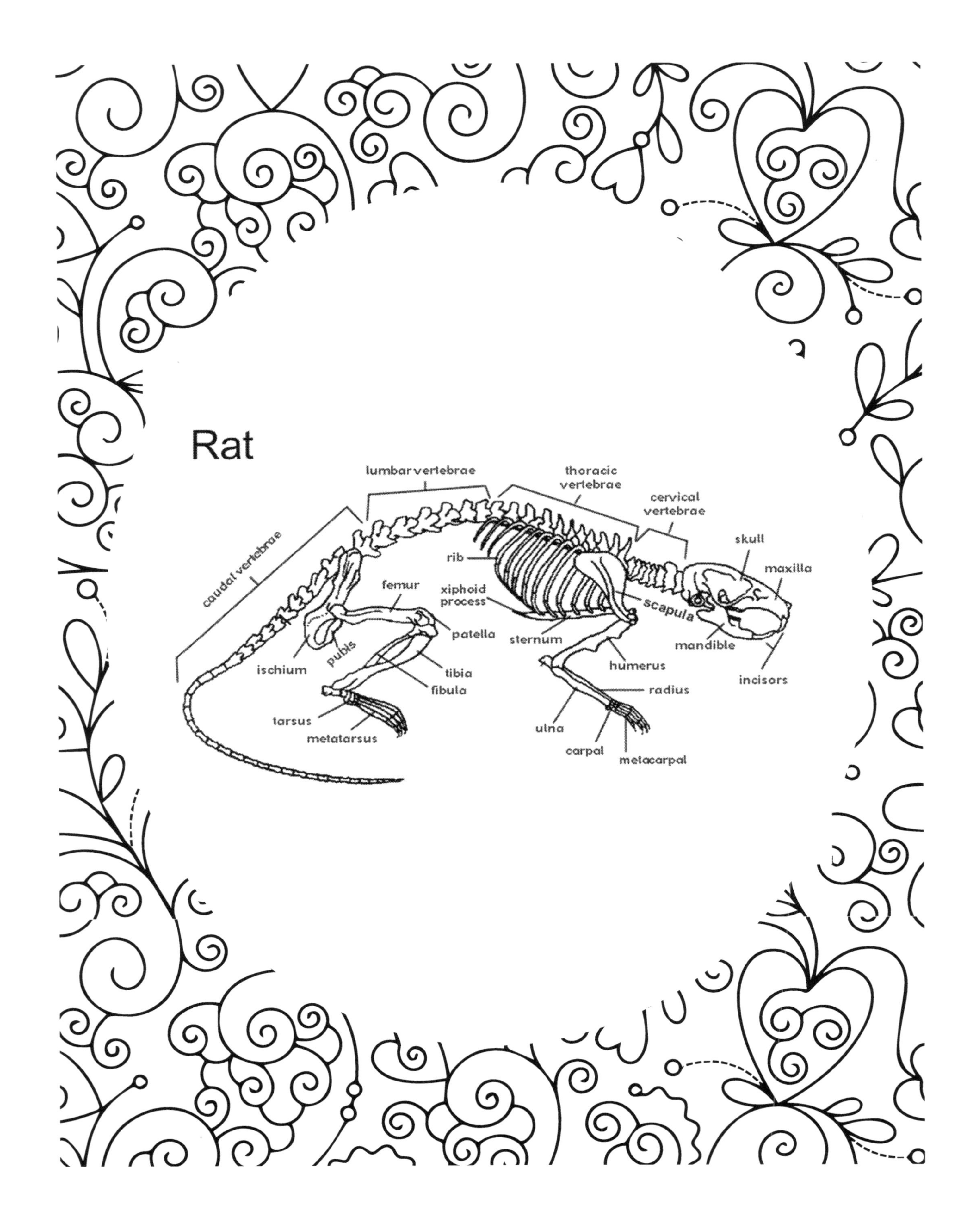
Rat
lumbar vertebrae
thoracic vertebrae
cervical vertebrae
caudal vertebrae
skull
maxilla
rib
femur
xiphoid process
scapula
patella
sternum
mandible
pubis
ischium
tibia
humerus
incisors
fibula
radius
tarsus
metatarsus
ulna
carpal
metacarpal

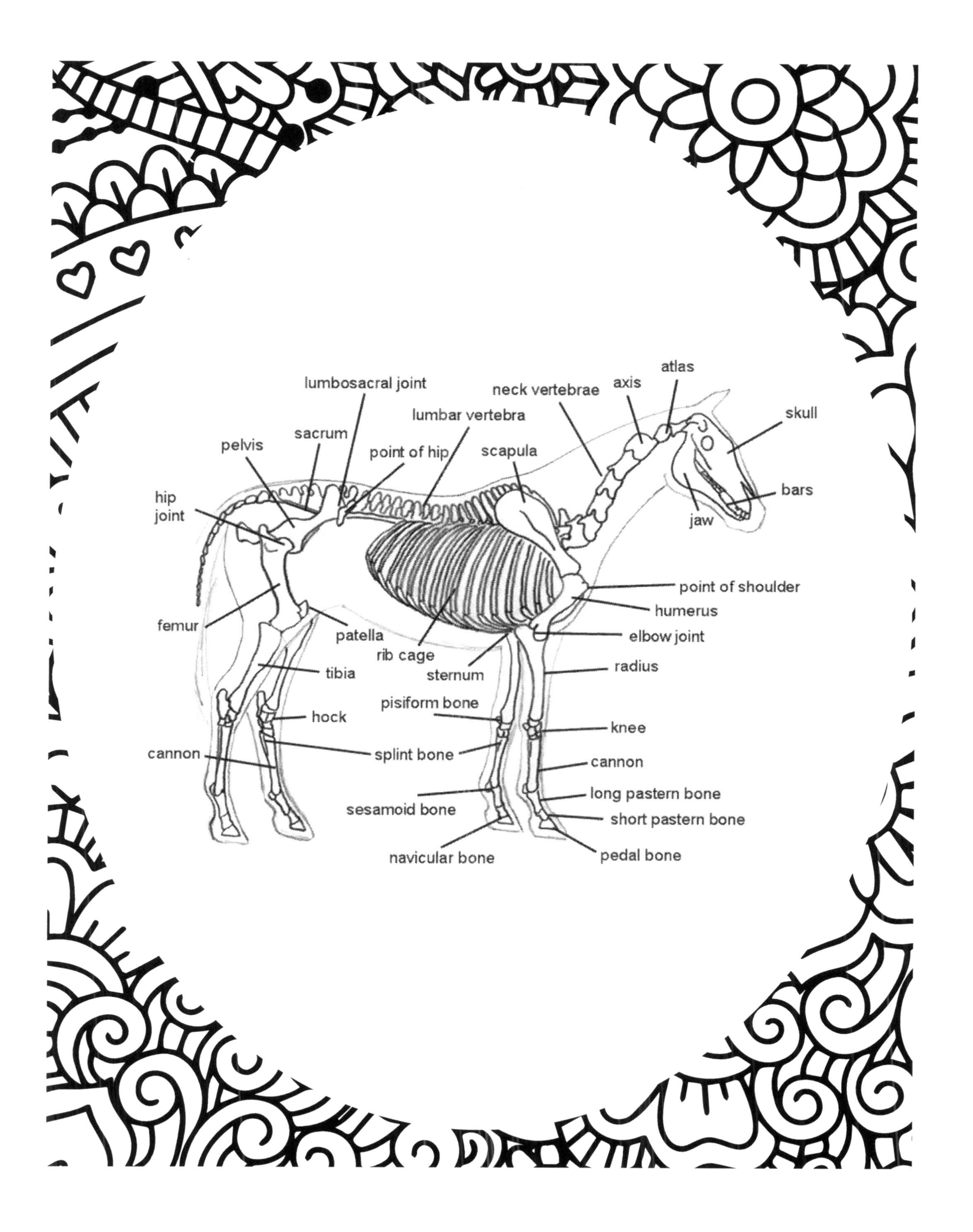
lumbosacral joint
atlas
neck vertebrae
axis
lumbar vertebra
skull
sacrum
pelvis
point of hip
scapula
hip
joint
bars
jaw
point of shoulder
humerus
femur
patella
elbow joint
rib cage
sternum
radius
tibia
pisiform bone
hock
knee
cannon
splint bone
cannon
long pastern bone
sesamoid bone
short pastern bone
pedal bone
navicular bone

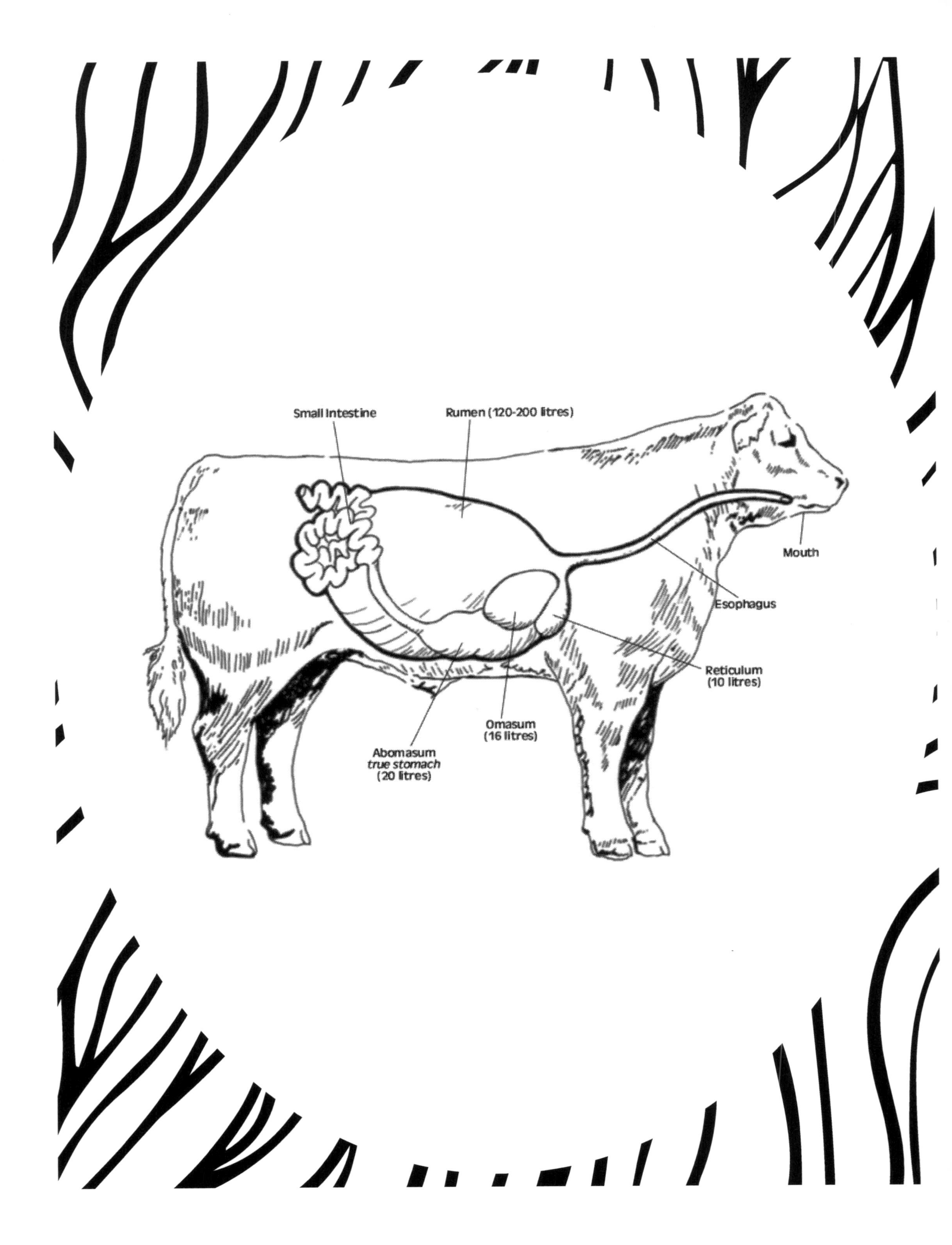
Small Intestine
Rumen (120-200 litres)
Mouth
Esophagus
Reticulum
(10 litres)
Omasum
(16 litres)
Abomasum
true stomach
(20 litres)

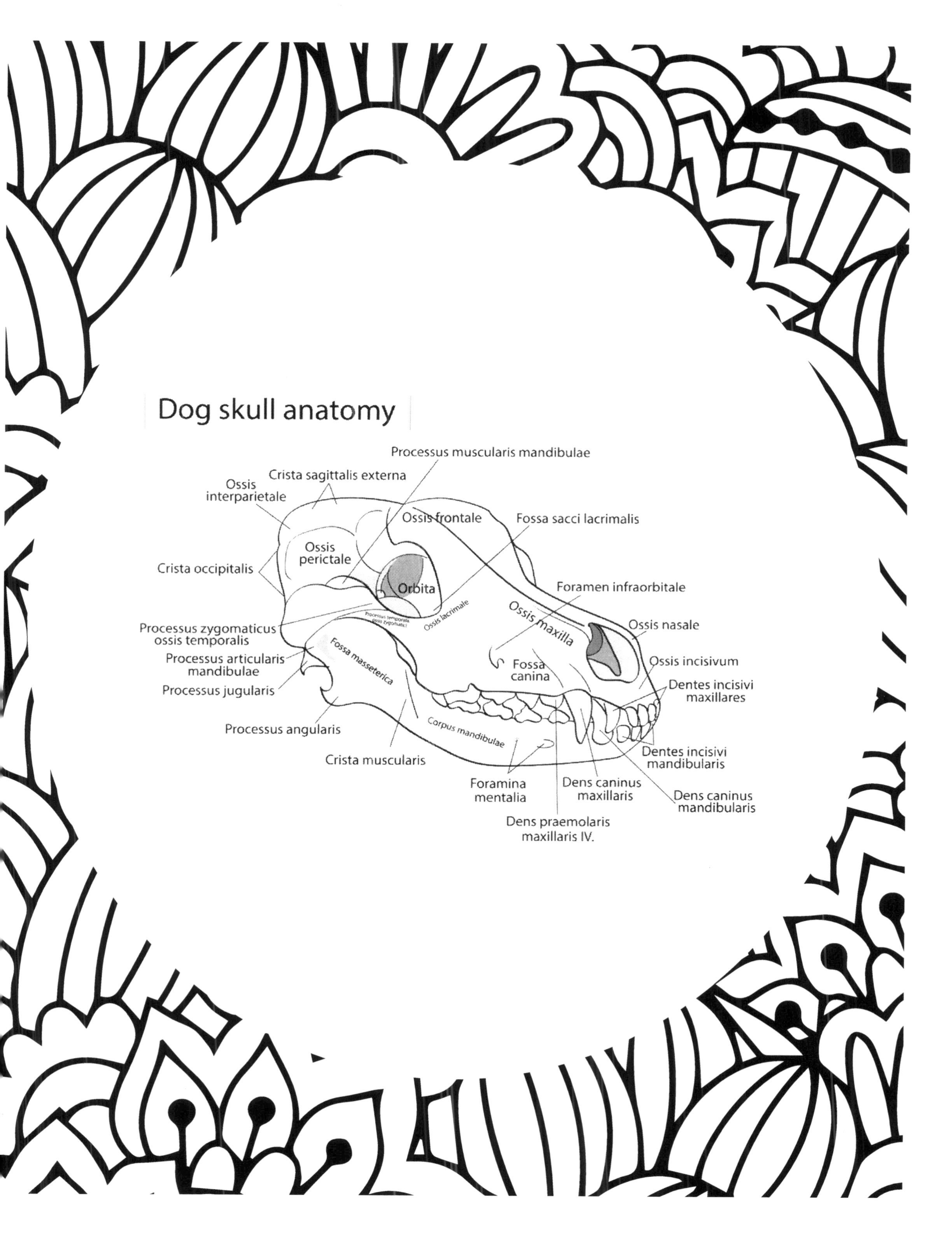
Dog skull anatomy
Processus muscularis mandibulae
Crista sagittalis externa
Ossis interparietale
Ossis frontale
Fossa sacci lacrimalis
Ossis perictale
Crista occipitalis
Orbita
Foramen infraorbitale
Ossis lacrimale
Ossis maxilla
Ossis nasale
Processus zygomaticus ossis temporalis
Fossa masseterica
Processus articularis mandibulae
Fossa canina
Ossis incisivum
Processus jugularis
Dentes incisivi maxillares
Corpus mandibulae
Processus angularis
Dentes incisivi mandibularis
Crista muscularis
Foramina mentalia
Dens caninus maxillaris
Dens caninus mandibularis
Dens praemolaris maxillaris IV.

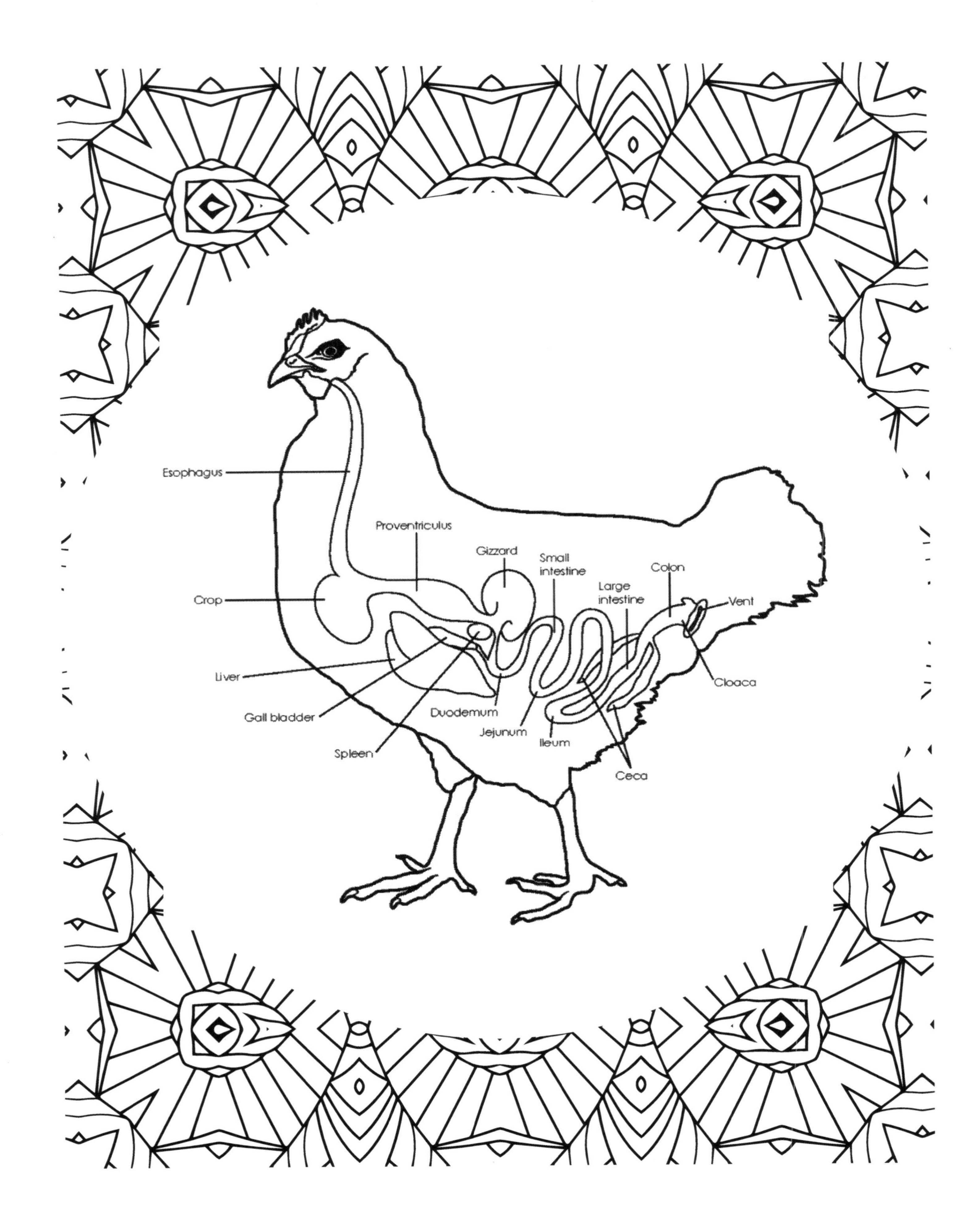
Esophagus
Proventriculus
Gizzard
Small intestine
Colon
Large intestine
Vent
Crop
Liver
Cloaca
Gall bladder
Duodemum
Jejunum
Ileum
Spleen
Ceca

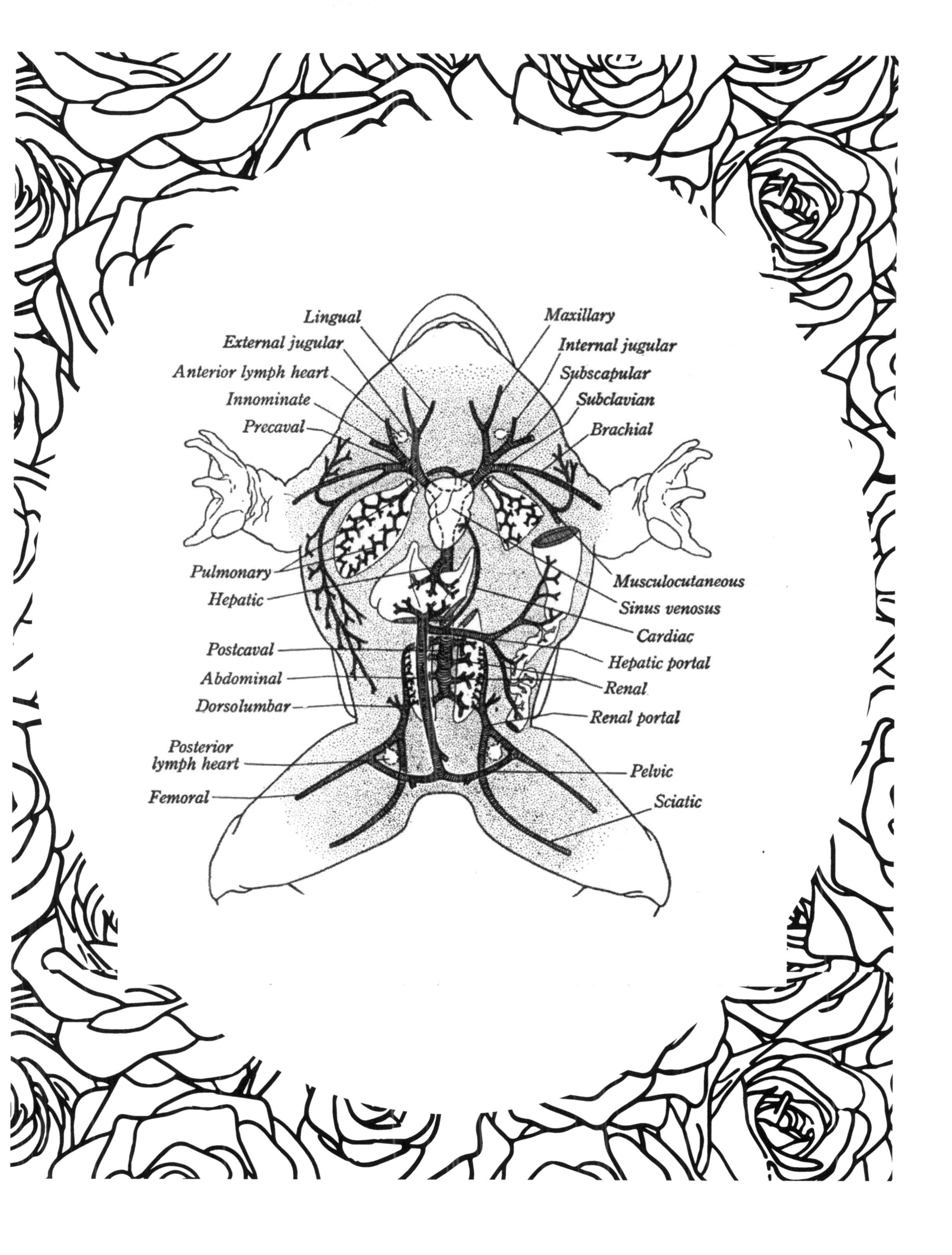
Lingual
External jugular
Anterior lymph heart
Innominate
Precaval
Pulmonary
Hepatic
Postcaval
Abdominal
Dorsolumbar
Posterior lymph heart
Femoral
Maxillary
Internal jugular
Subscapular
Subclavian
Brachial
Musculocutaneous
Sinus venosus
Cardiac
Hepatic portal
Renal
Renal portal
Pelvic
Sciatic

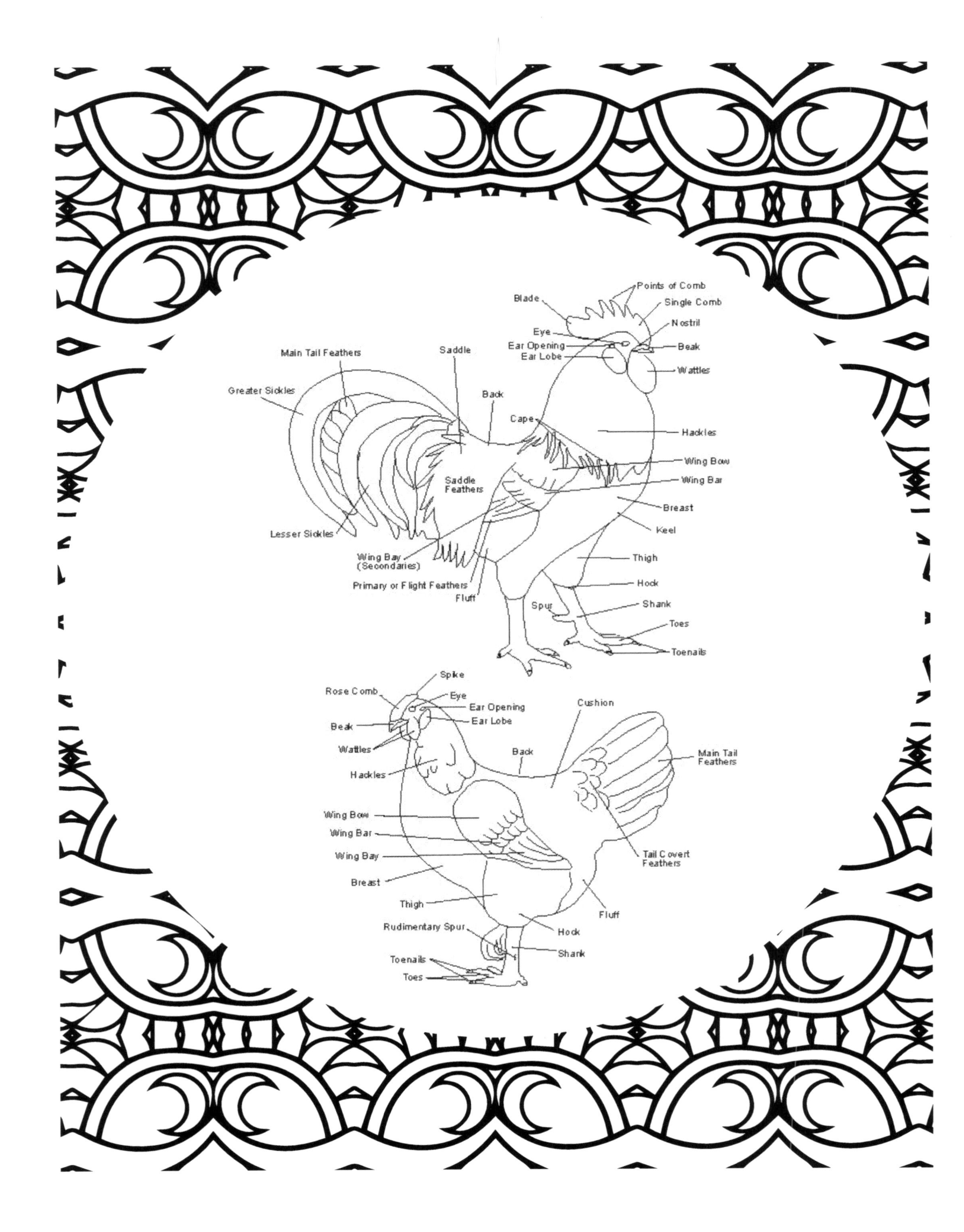
Points of Comb
Blade
Single Comb
Nostril
Eye
Ear Opening
Beak
Ear Lobe
Wattles
Main Tail Feathers
Saddle
Greater Sickles
Back
Cape
Hackles
Wing Bow
Wing Bar
Saddle Feathers
Breast
Keel
Lesser Sickles
Wing Bay (Secondaries)
Thigh
Primary or Flight Feathers
Hock
Fluff
Spur
Shank
Toes
Toenails
Spike
Rose Comb
Eye
Ear Opening
Cushion
Ear Lobe
Beak
Wattles
Back
Main Tail Feathers
Hackles
Wing Bow
Wing Bar
Wing Bay
Tail Covert Feathers
Breast
Thigh
Fluff
Rudimentary Spur
Hock
Shank
Toenails
Toes

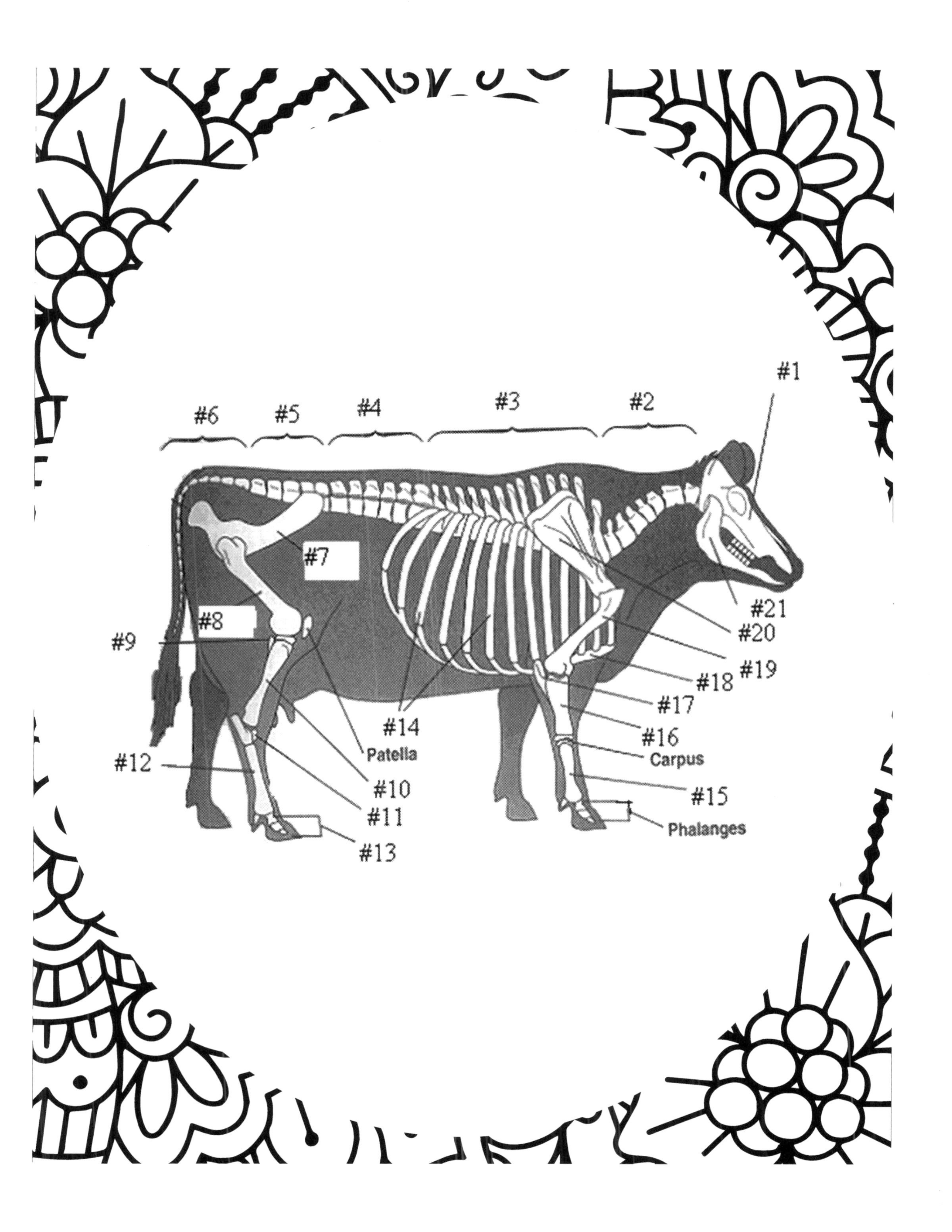
#1
#2
#3
#4
#5
#6
#7
#8
#9
#10
#11
#12
#13
#14
#15
#16
#17
#18
#19
#20
#21
Patella
Carpus
Phalanges

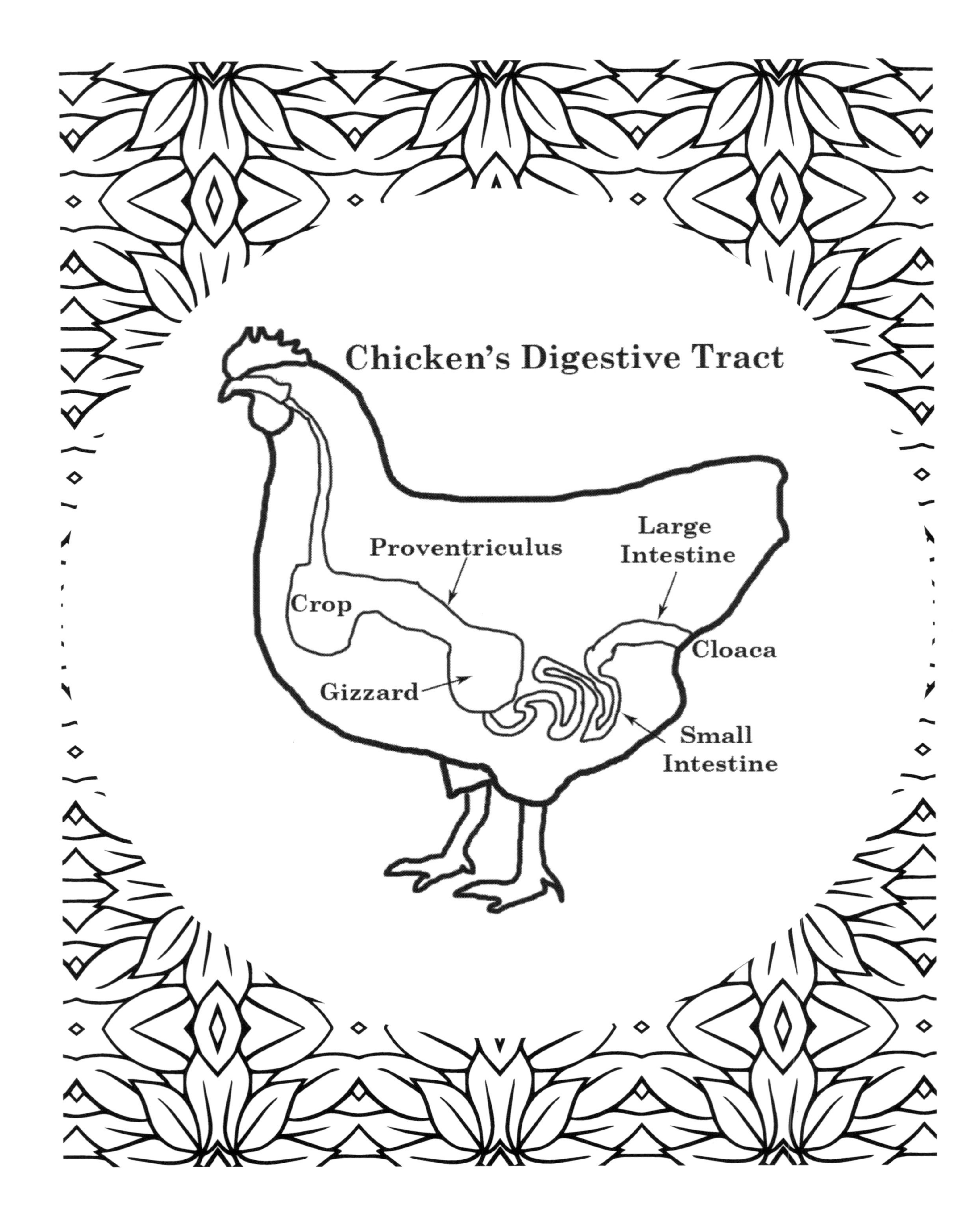

Chicken's Digestive Tract
Proventriculus
Large
Intestine
Crop
Cloaca
Gizzard
Small
Intestine

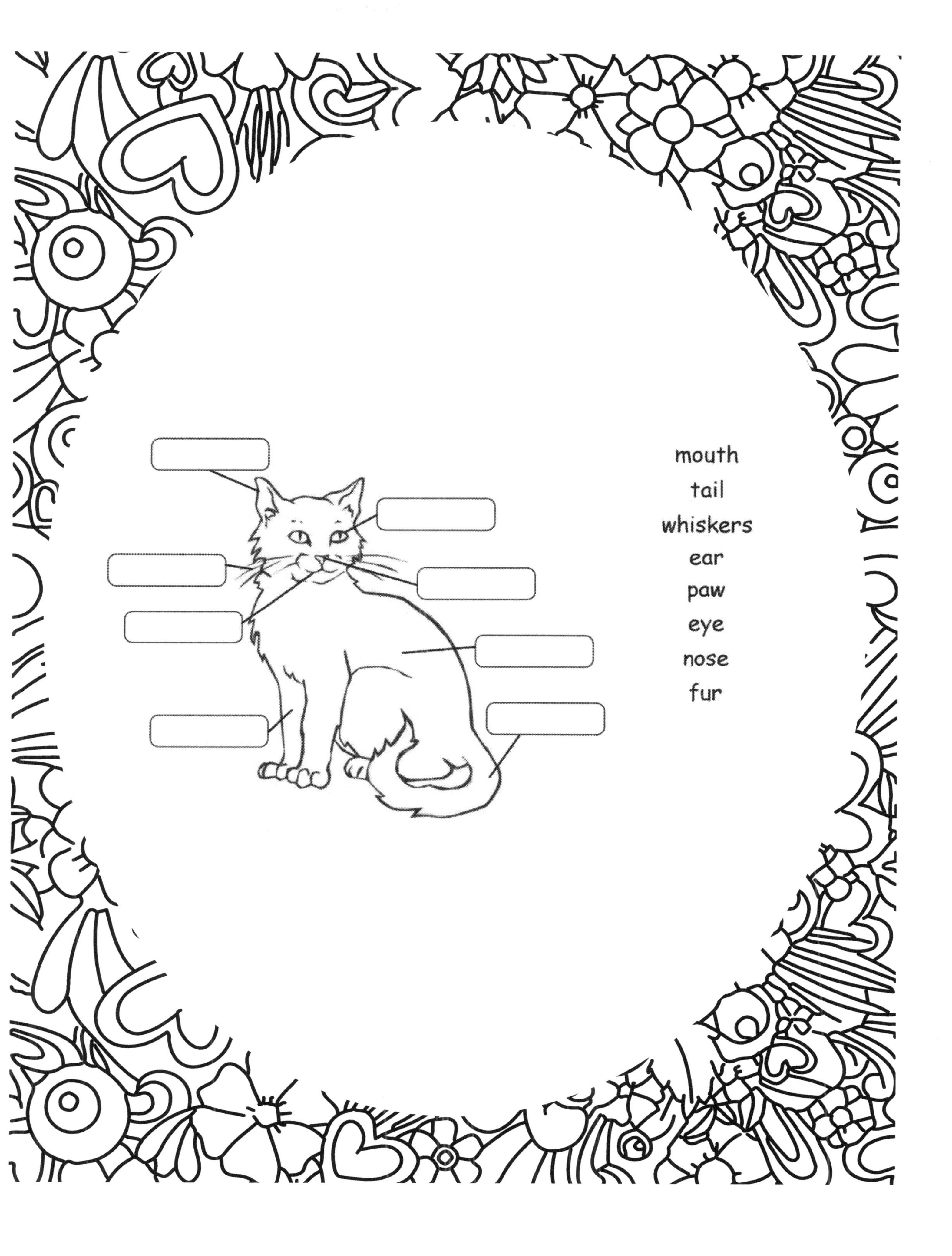
mouth
tail
whiskers
ear
paw
eye
nose
fur

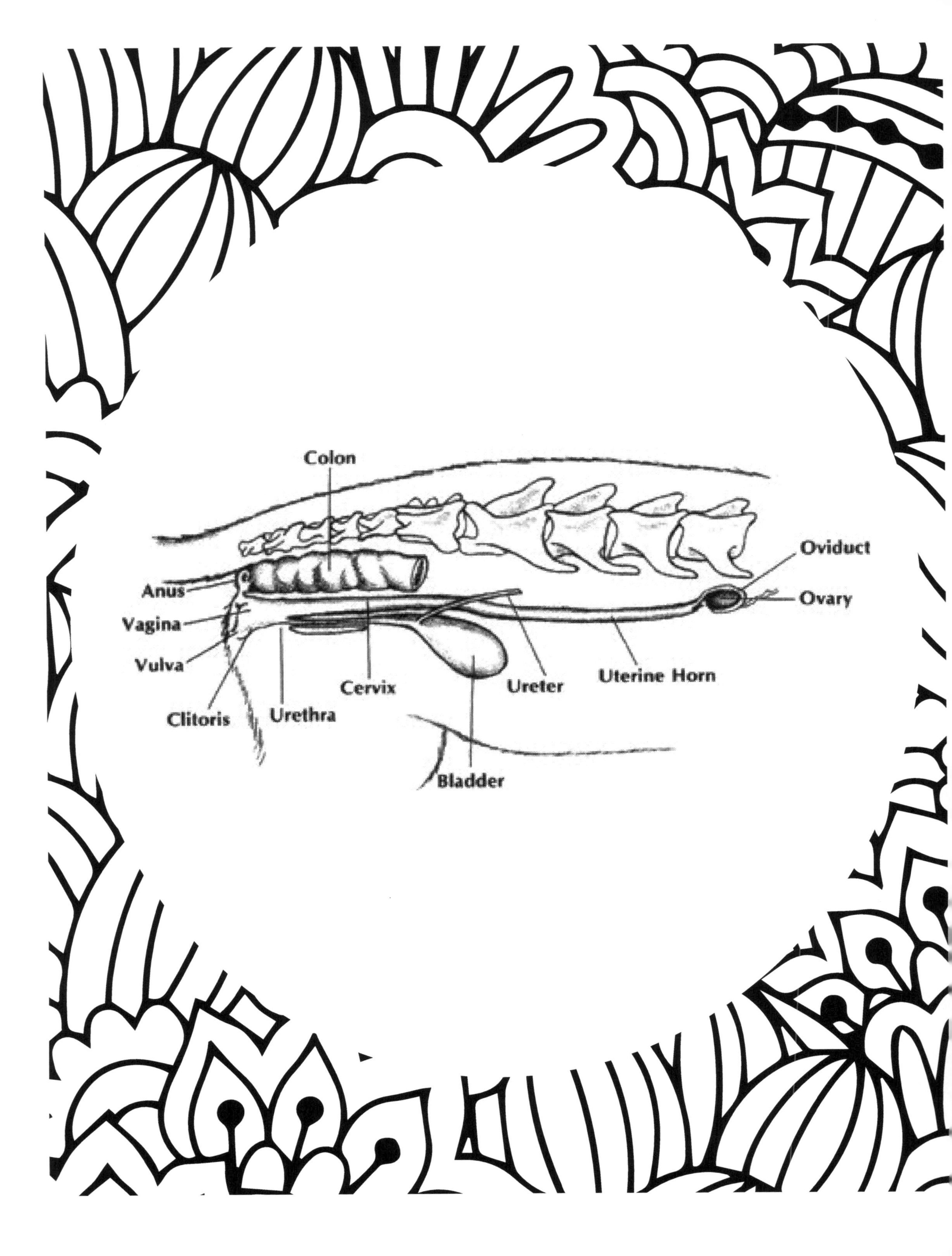
Colon
Oviduct
Anus
Ovary
Vagina
Vulva
Cervix
Ureter
Uterine Horn
Clitoris
Urethra
Bladder

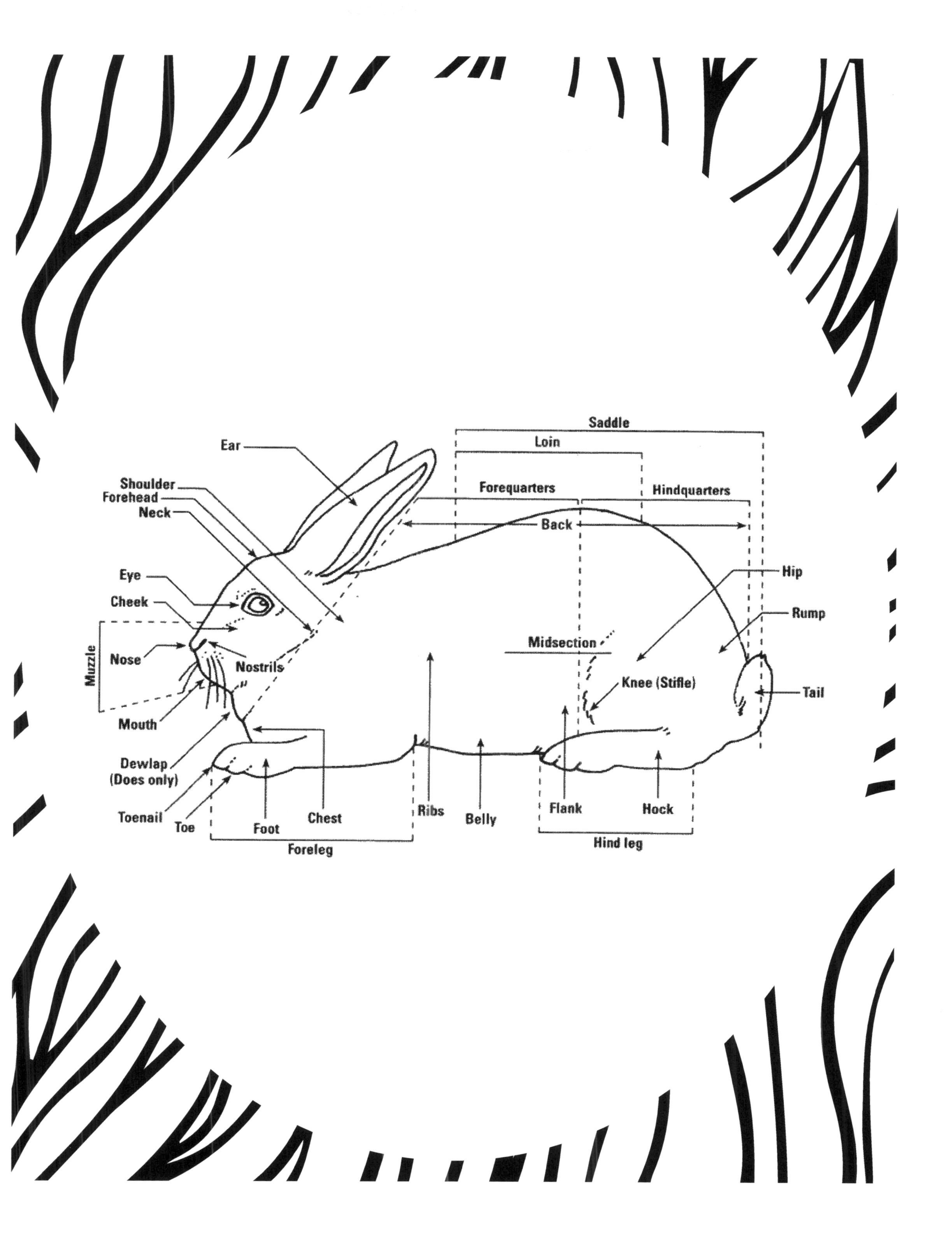
Saddle
Loin
Forequarters
Hindquarters
Ear
Shoulder
Forehead
Neck
Back
Eye
Cheek
Hip
Rump
Muzzle
Nose
Nostrils
Midsection
Knee (Stifle)
Tail
Mouth
Dewlap
(Does only)
Toenail
Toe
Foot
Chest
Ribs
Belly
Flank
Hock
Foreleg
Hind leg

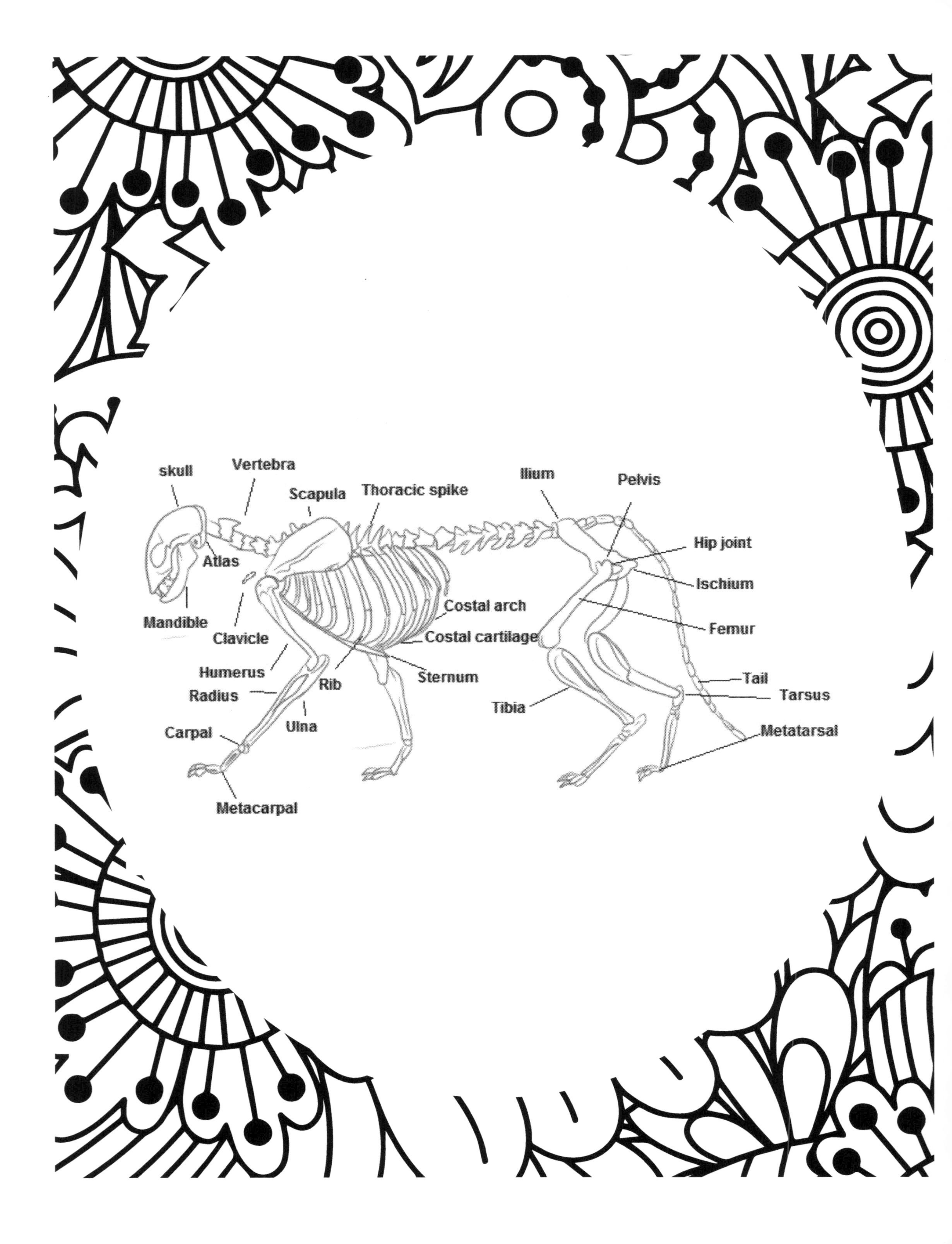
skull
Vertebra
Scapula
Thoracic spike
Ilium
Pelvis
Atlas
Hip joint
Ischium
Costal arch
Mandible
Clavicle
Costal cartilage
Femur
Humerus
Sternum
Rib
Radius
Tail
Tarsus
Tibia
Ulna
Carpal
Metatarsal
Metacarpal

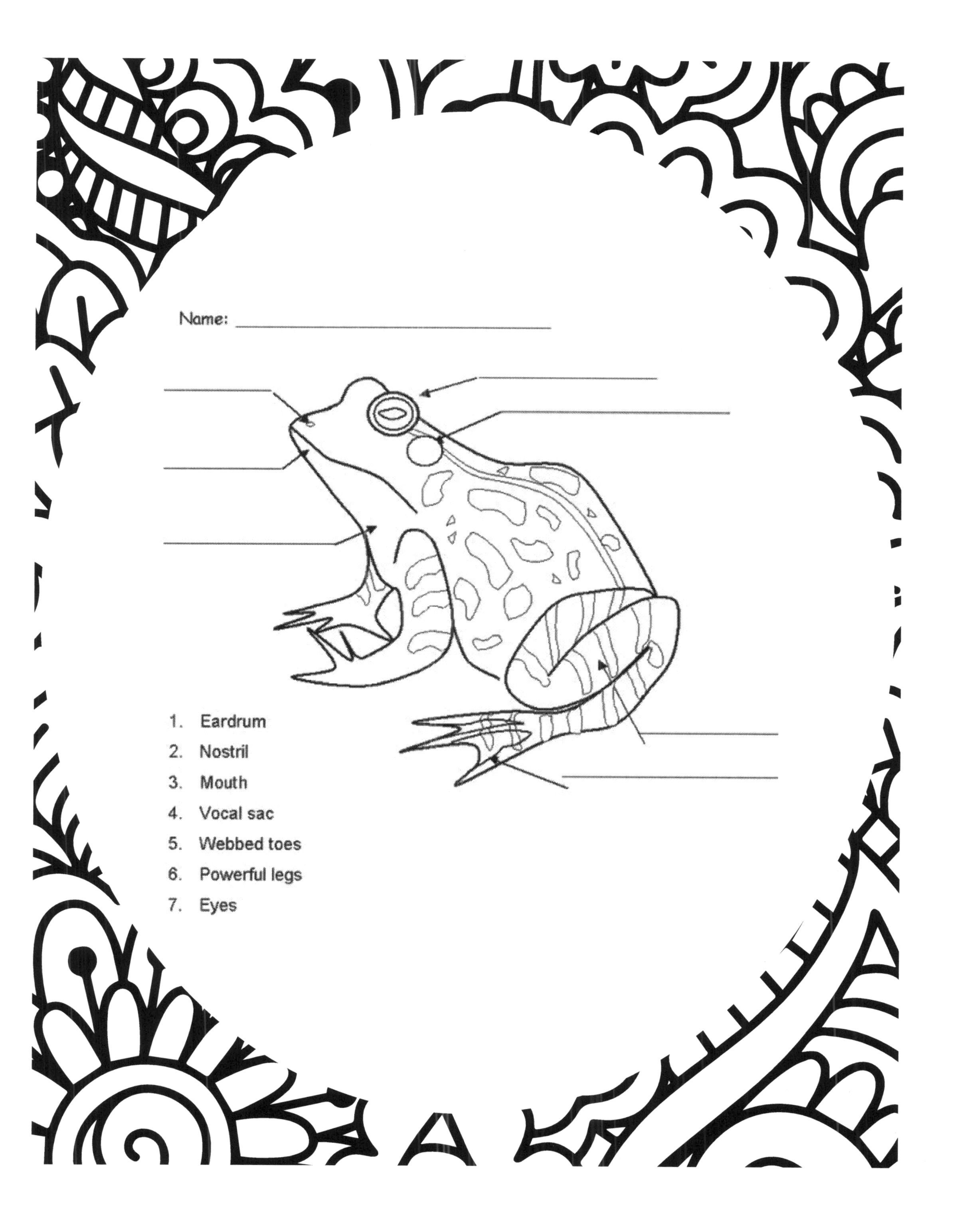
Name:
1. Eardrum
2. Nostril
3. Mouth
4. Vocal sac
5. Webbed toes
6. Powerful legs
7. Eyes

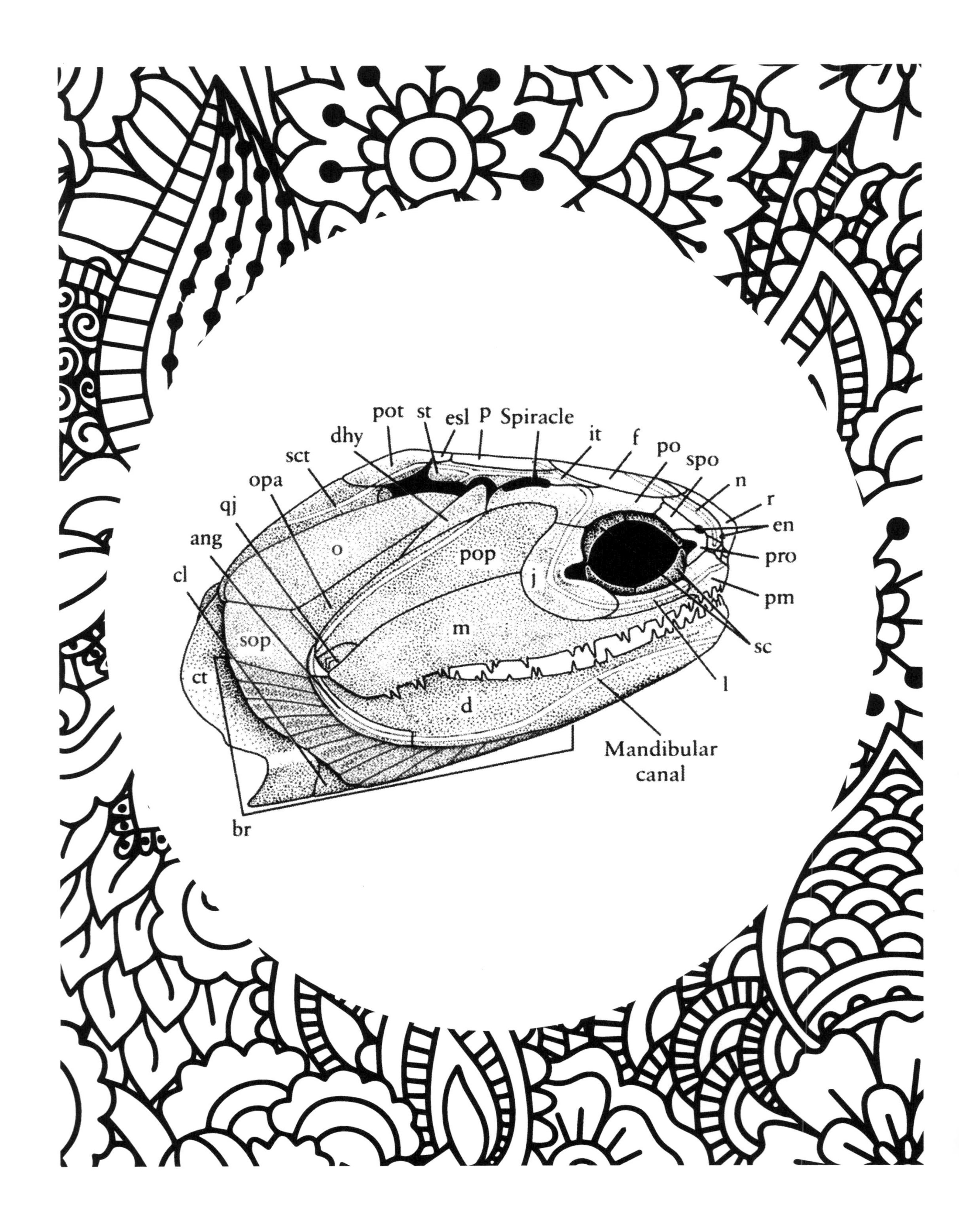
pot
st
esl
P
Spiracle
it
f
po
spo
dhy
sct
opa
qj
ang
cl
n
r
en
pro
pm
o
pop
j
m
sop
ct
d
sc
l
Mandibular
canal
br

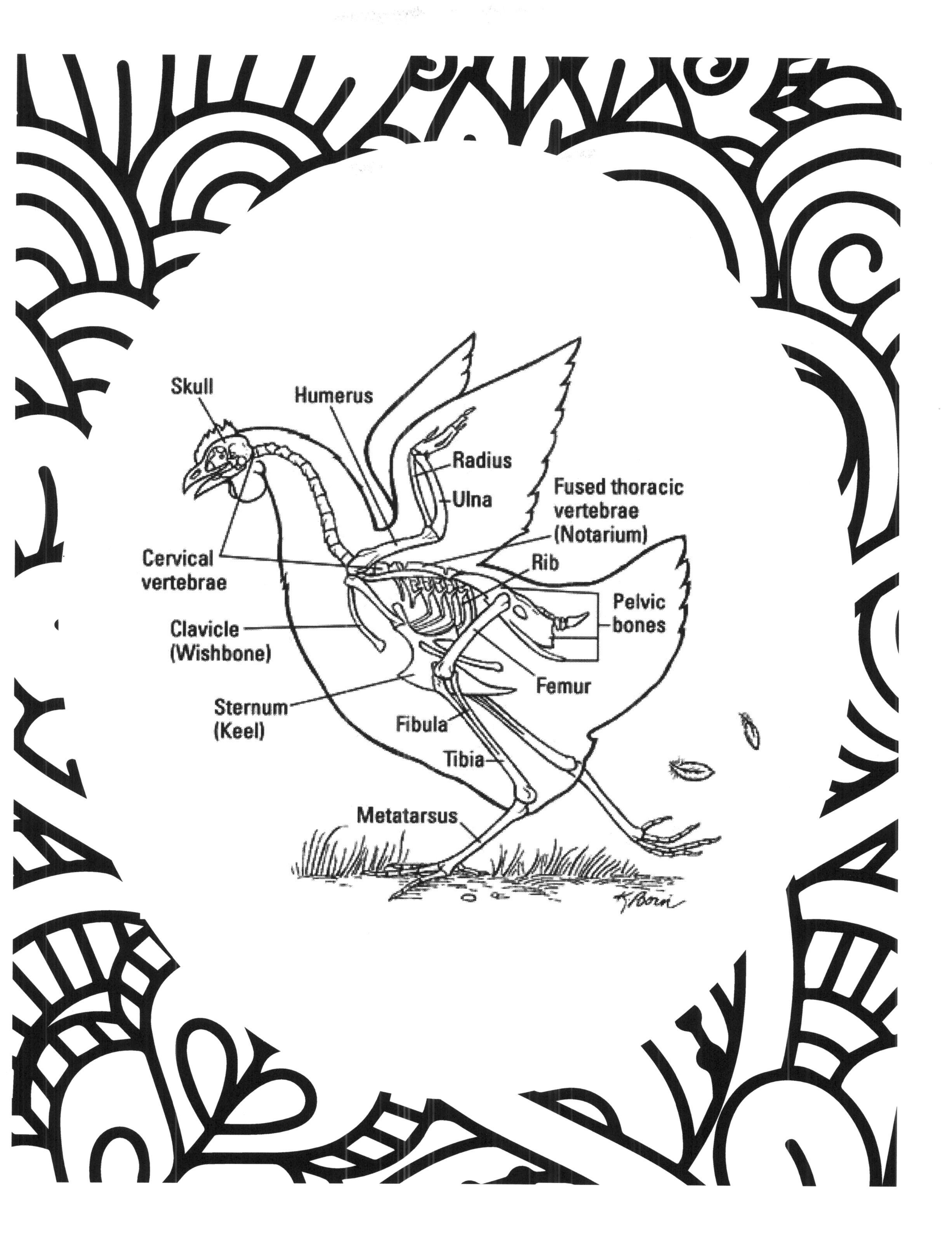
Skull
Humerus
Radius
Ulna
Fused thoracic vertebrae (Notarium)
Rib
Cervical vertebrae
Pelvic bones
Clavicle (Wishbone)
Femur
Sternum (Keel)
Fibula
Tibia
Metatarsus

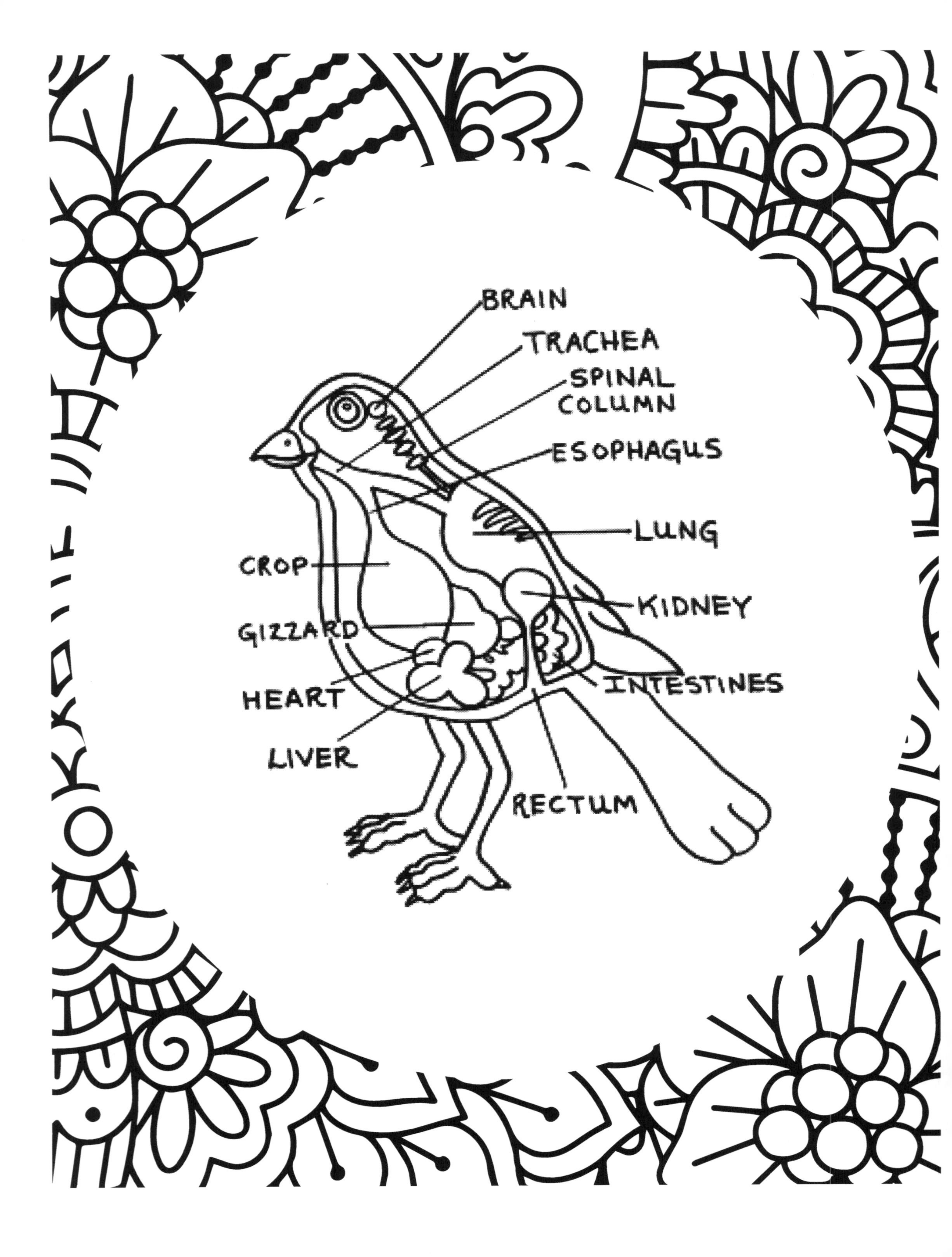
BRAIN
TRACHEA
SPINAL COLUMN
ESOPHAGUS
LUNG
CROP
KIDNEY
GIZZARD
INTESTINES
HEART
LIVER
RECTUM

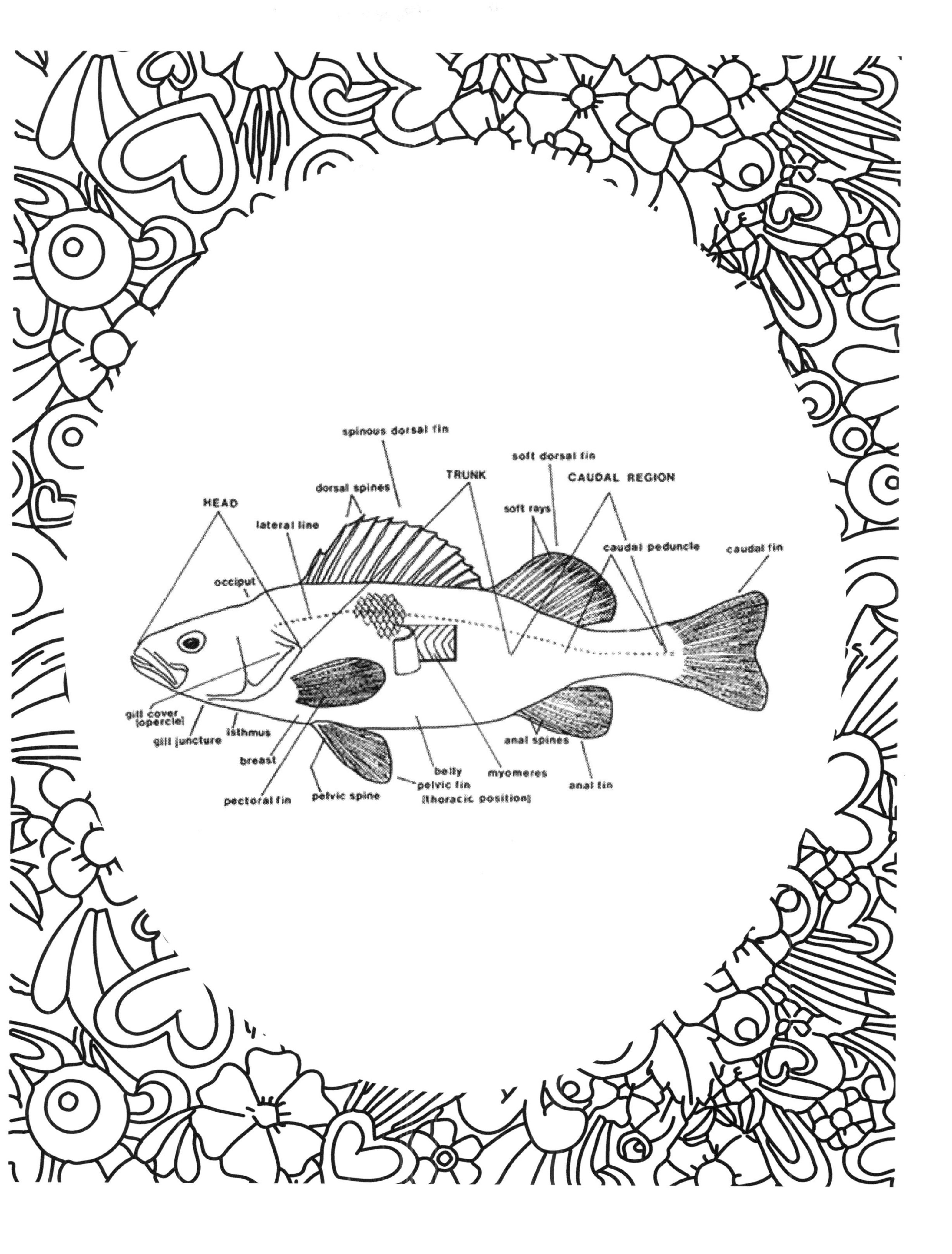
spinous dorsal fin
soft dorsal fin
TRUNK
CAUDAL REGION
dorsal spines
HEAD
lateral line
soft rays
caudal peduncle
caudal fin
occiput
gill cover
(opercle)
gill juncture
isthmus
breast
pectoral fin
pelvic spine
belly
pelvic fin
(thoracic position)
myomeres
anal spines
anal fin

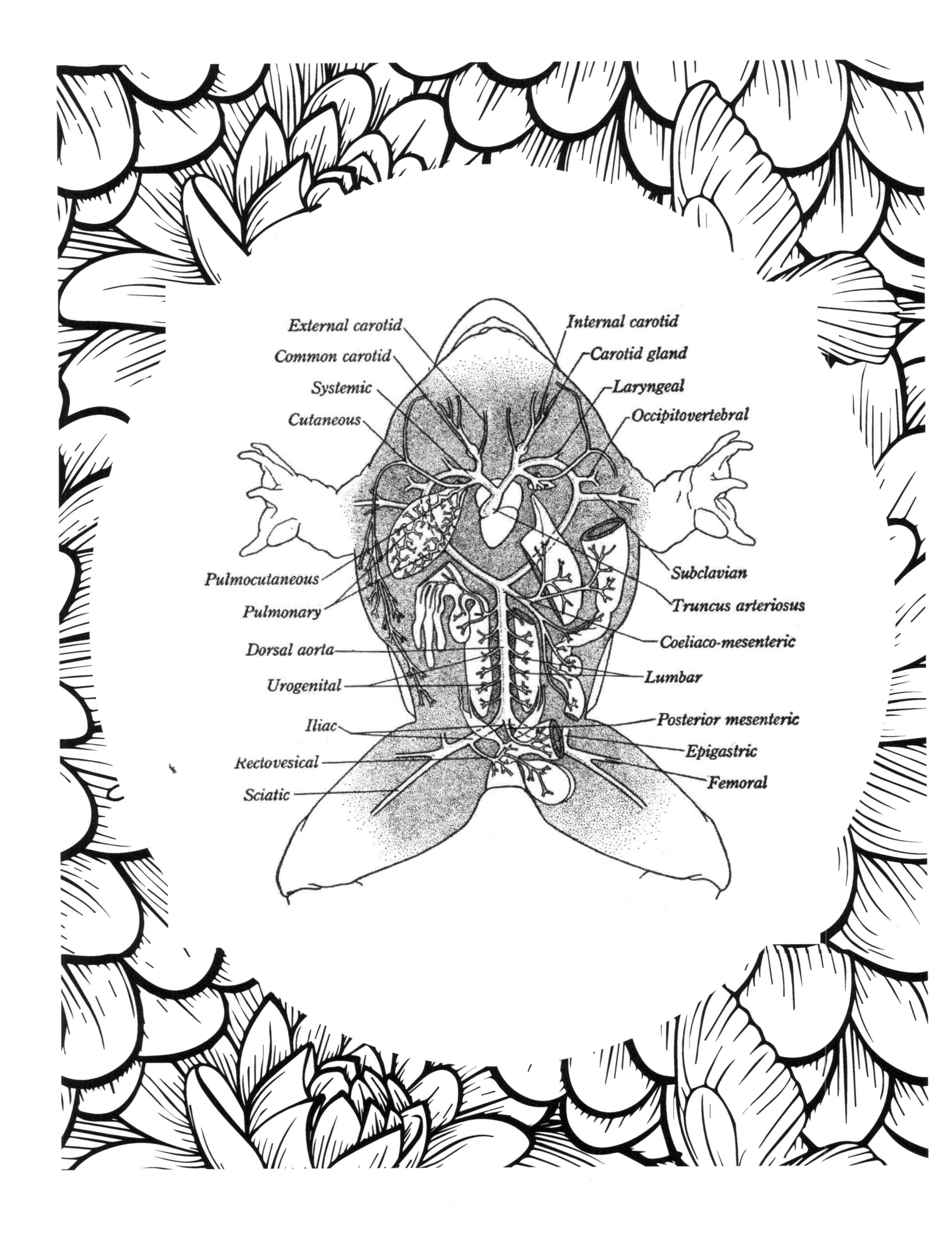
External carotid
Internal carotid
Common carotid
Carotid gland
Systemic
Laryngeal
Cutaneous
Occipitovertebral
Subclavian
Pulmocutaneous
Truncus arteriosus
Pulmonary
Coeliaco-mesenteric
Dorsal aorta
Lumbar
Urogenital
Posterior mesenteric
Iliac
Epigastric
Rectovesical
Femoral
Sciatic

Anatomy of the Frog

esophagus
carotid artery
aortic arch
subclavian artery
lungs
liver
gall bladder
fat bodies
kidney
small intestine
mesentery
common iliac artery
femoral artery
sciatic artery
conus arteriosus of heart
stomach
pancreas
spleen
bladder
large intestine
cloaca

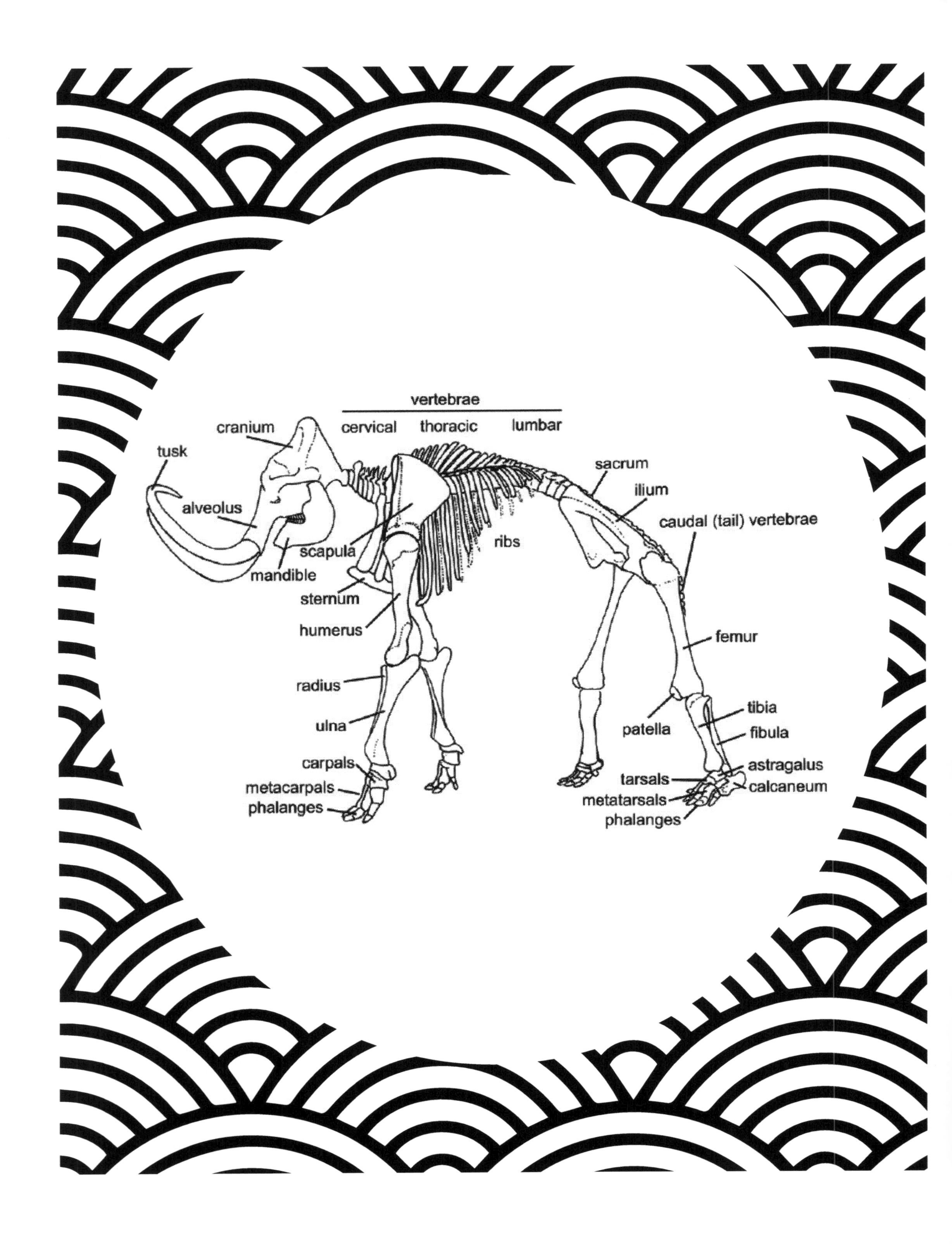
vertebrae
cervical
thoracic
lumbar
cranium
tusk
alveolus
scapula
mandible
sternum
humerus
radius
ulna
carpals
metacarpals
phalanges
ribs
sacrum
ilium
caudal (tail) vertebrae
femur
patella
tibia
fibula
astragalus
tarsals
calcaneum
metatarsals
phalanges

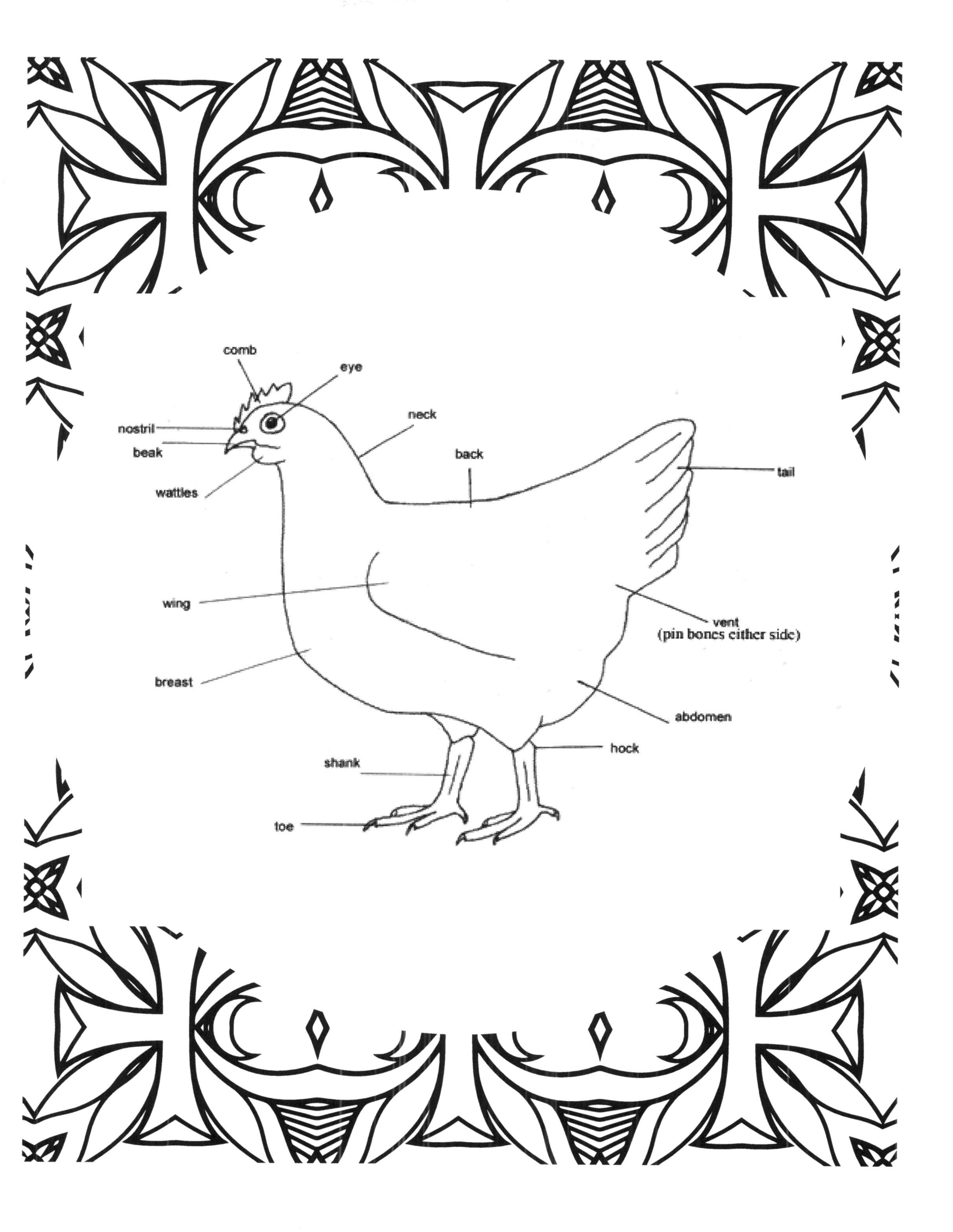
comb
eye
nostril
beak
neck
back
tail
wattles
wing
vent
(pin bones either side)
breast
abdomen
hock
shank
toe

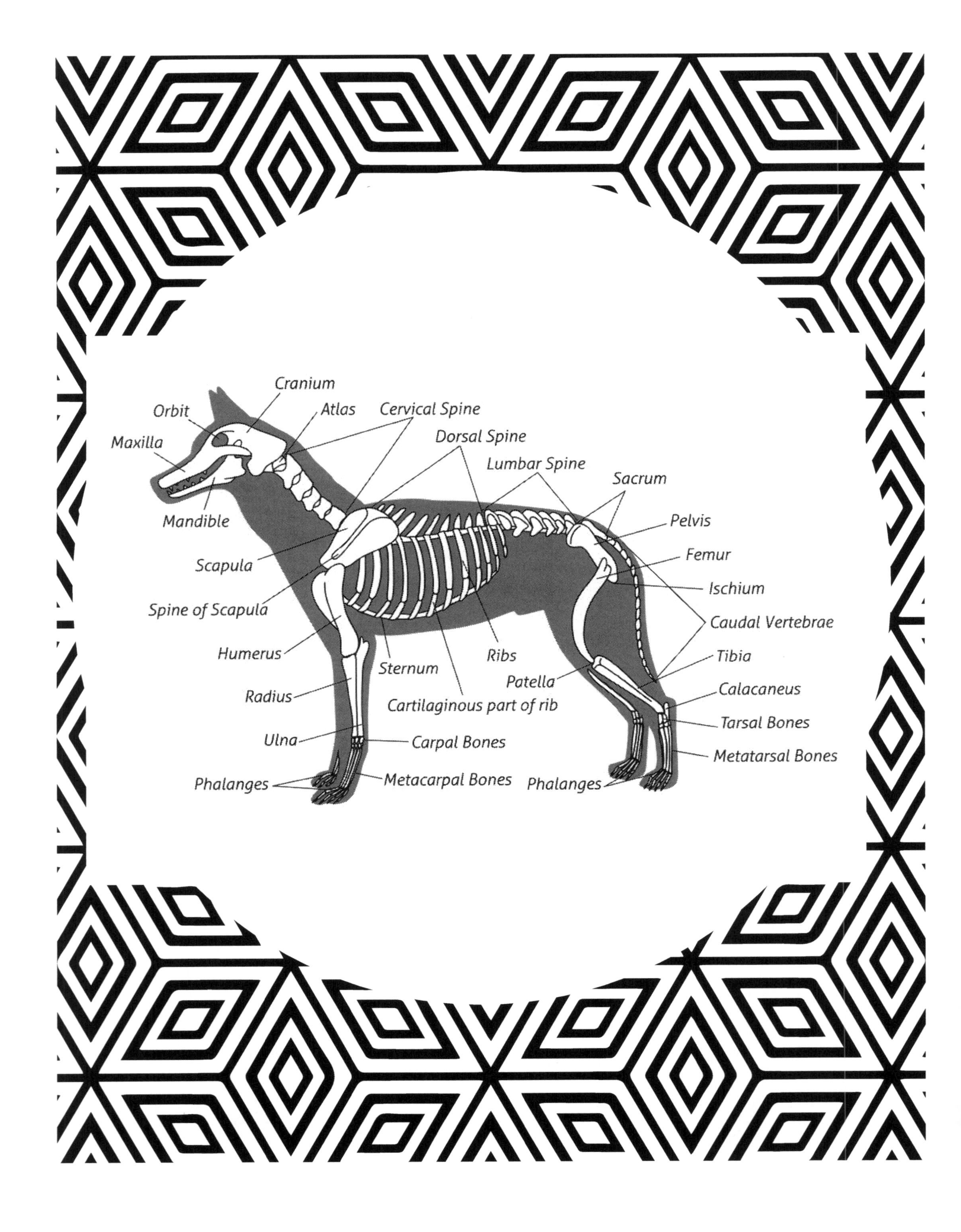
Cranium
Orbit
Atlas
Cervical Spine
Maxilla
Dorsal Spine
Lumbar Spine
Sacrum
Mandible
Pelvis
Scapula
Femur
Ischium
Spine of Scapula
Caudal Vertebrae
Humerus
Ribs
Tibia
Sternum
Patella
Radius
Calacaneus
Cartilaginous part of rib
Tarsal Bones
Ulna
Carpal Bones
Metatarsal Bones
Phalanges
Metacarpal Bones
Phalanges

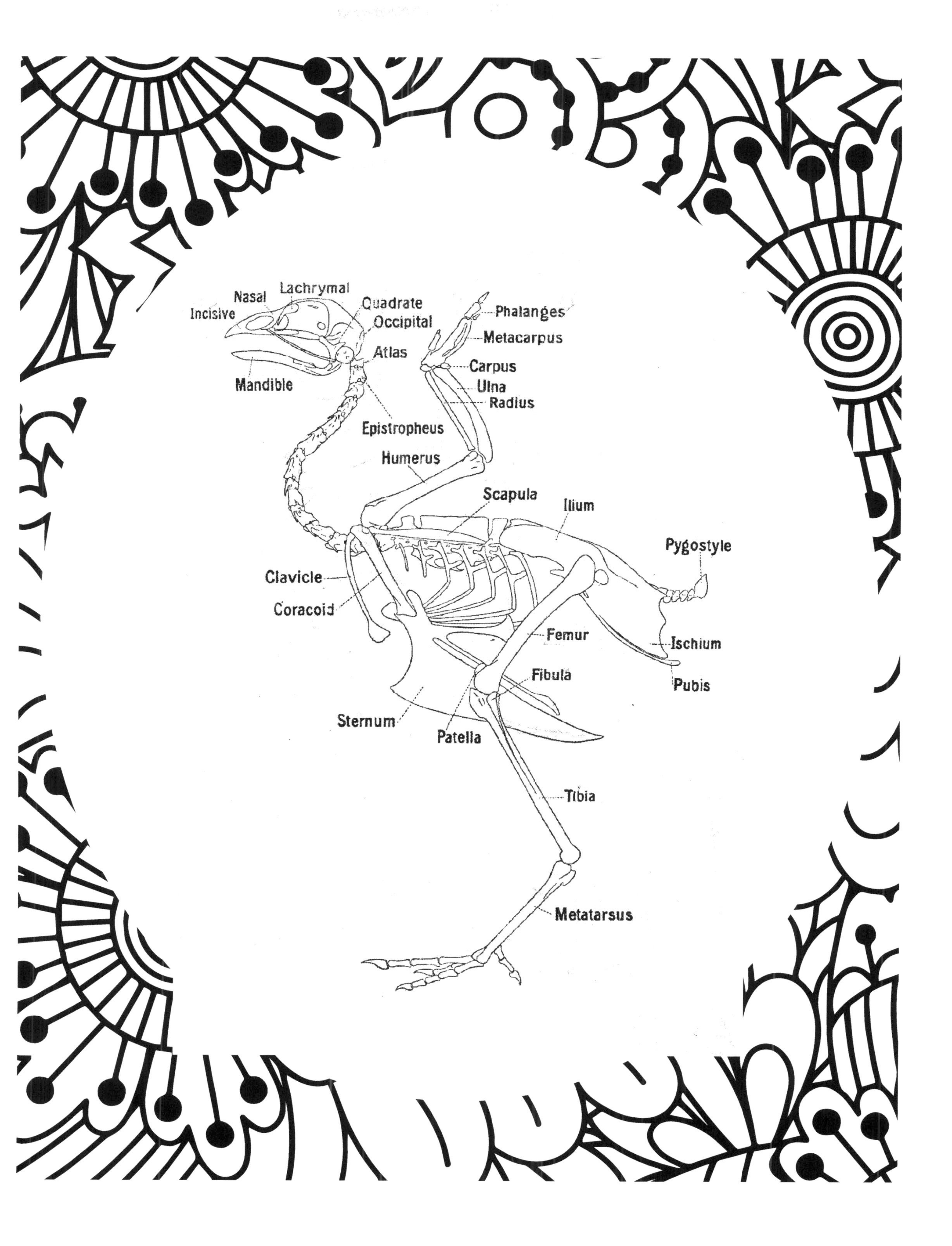

Incisive
Nasal
Lachrymal
Quadrate
Occipital
Phalanges
Metacarpus
Atlas
Mandible
Carpus
Ulna
Radius
Epistropheus
Humerus
Scapula
Ilium
Pygostyle
Clavicle
Coracoid
Femur
Ischium
Fibula
Pubis
Sternum
Patella
Tibia
Metatarsus

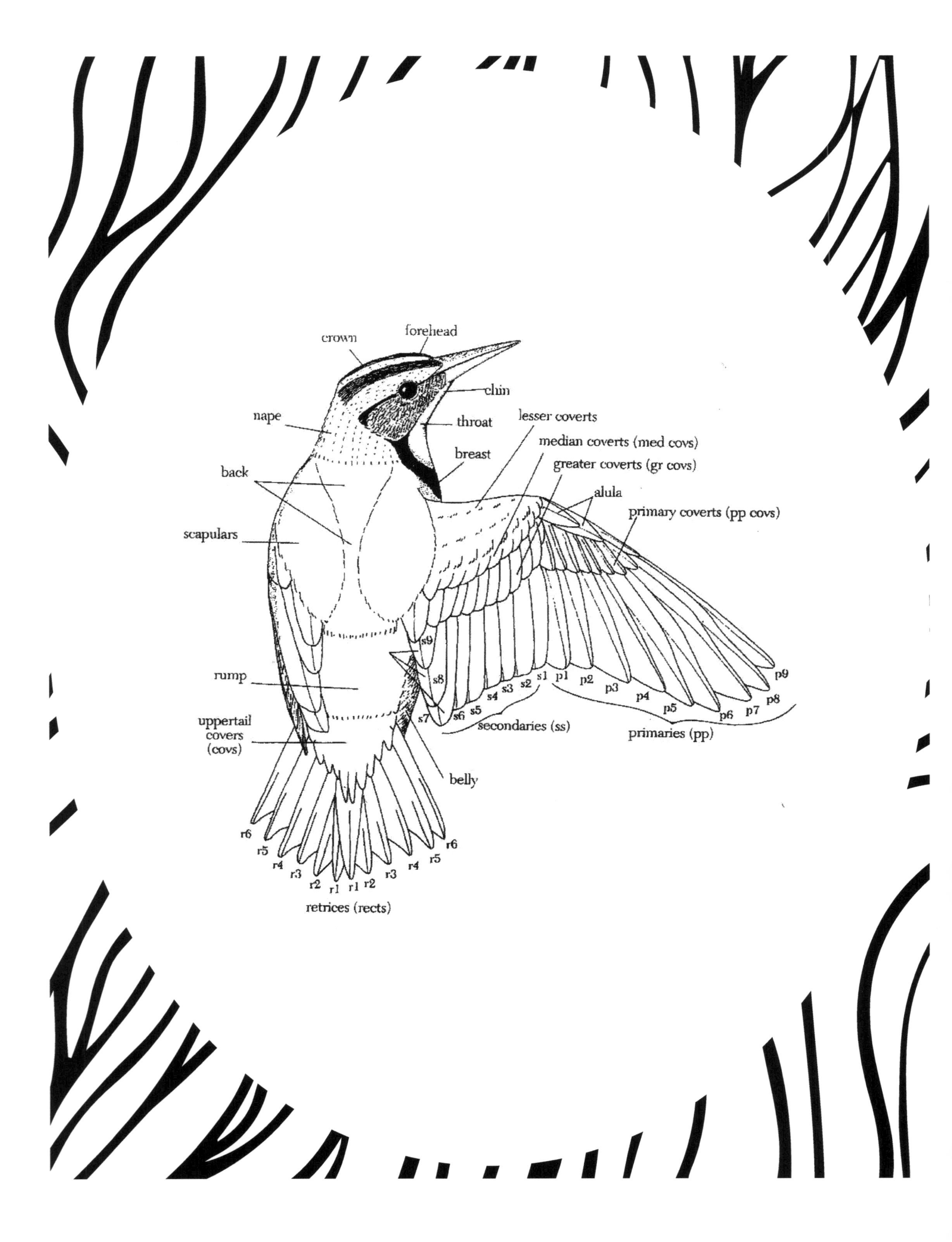
crown
forehead
chin
nape
throat
lesser coverts
median coverts (med covs)
breast
greater coverts (gr covs)
back
alula
primary coverts (pp covs)
scapulars
s9
rump
s8
s1 p1 p2 p3 p4 p5 p6 p7 p8 p9
s2 s3 s4 s5 s6 s7
uppertail
covers
(covs)
secondaries (ss)
primaries (pp)
belly
r6 r5 r4 r3 r2 r1 r1 r2 r3 r4 r5 r6
retrices (rects)

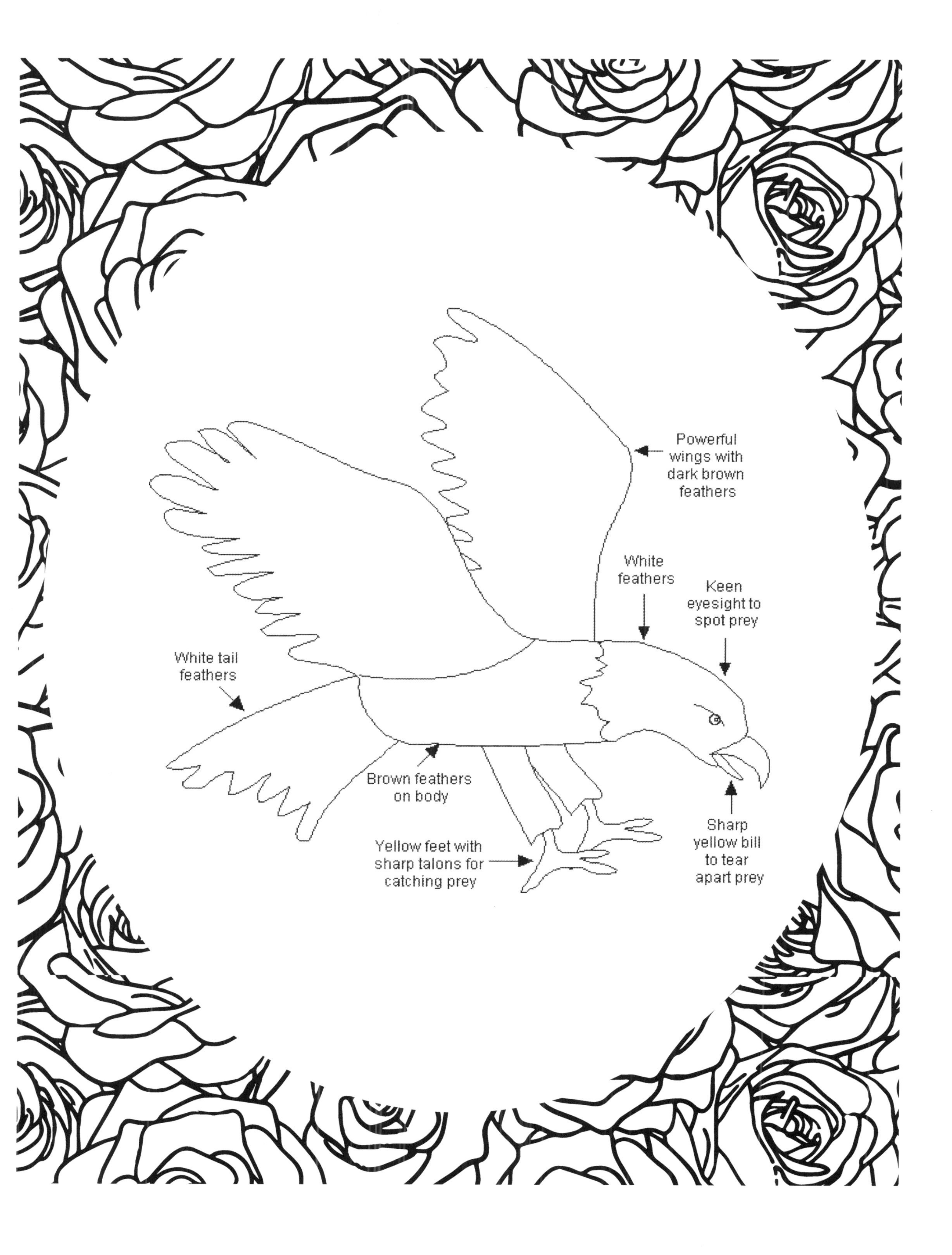

Powerful wings with dark brown feathers
White feathers
Keen eyesight to spot prey
White tail feathers
Brown feathers on body
Yellow feet with sharp talons for catching prey
Sharp yellow bill to tear apart prey

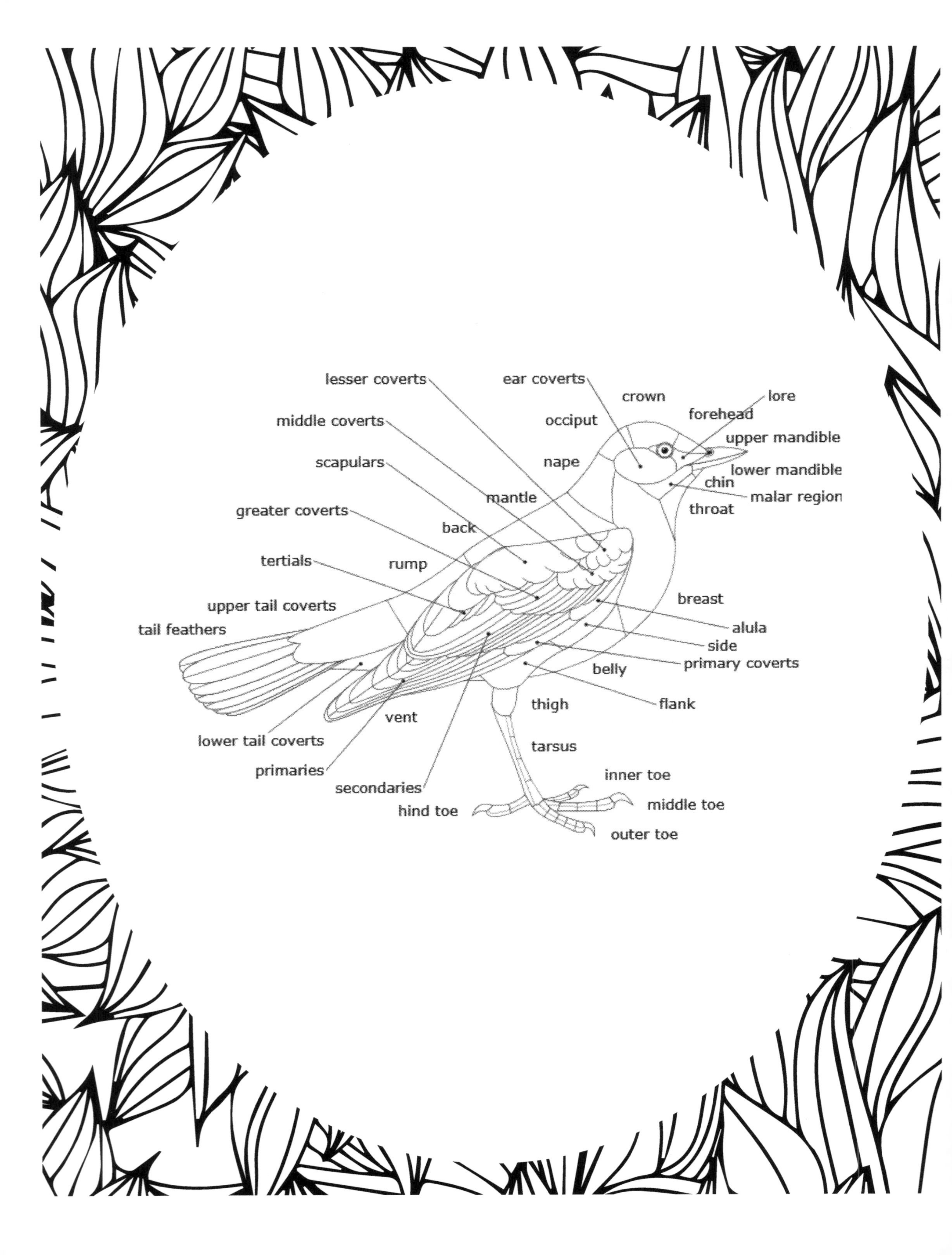
lesser coverts
ear coverts
crown
lore
forehead
middle coverts
occiput
upper mandible
scapulars
nape
lower mandible
chin
mantle
malar region
greater coverts
throat
back
tertials
rump
breast
upper tail coverts
alula
tail feathers
side
primary coverts
belly
flank
thigh
vent
lower tail coverts
tarsus
primaries
inner toe
secondaries
middle toe
hind toe
outer toe

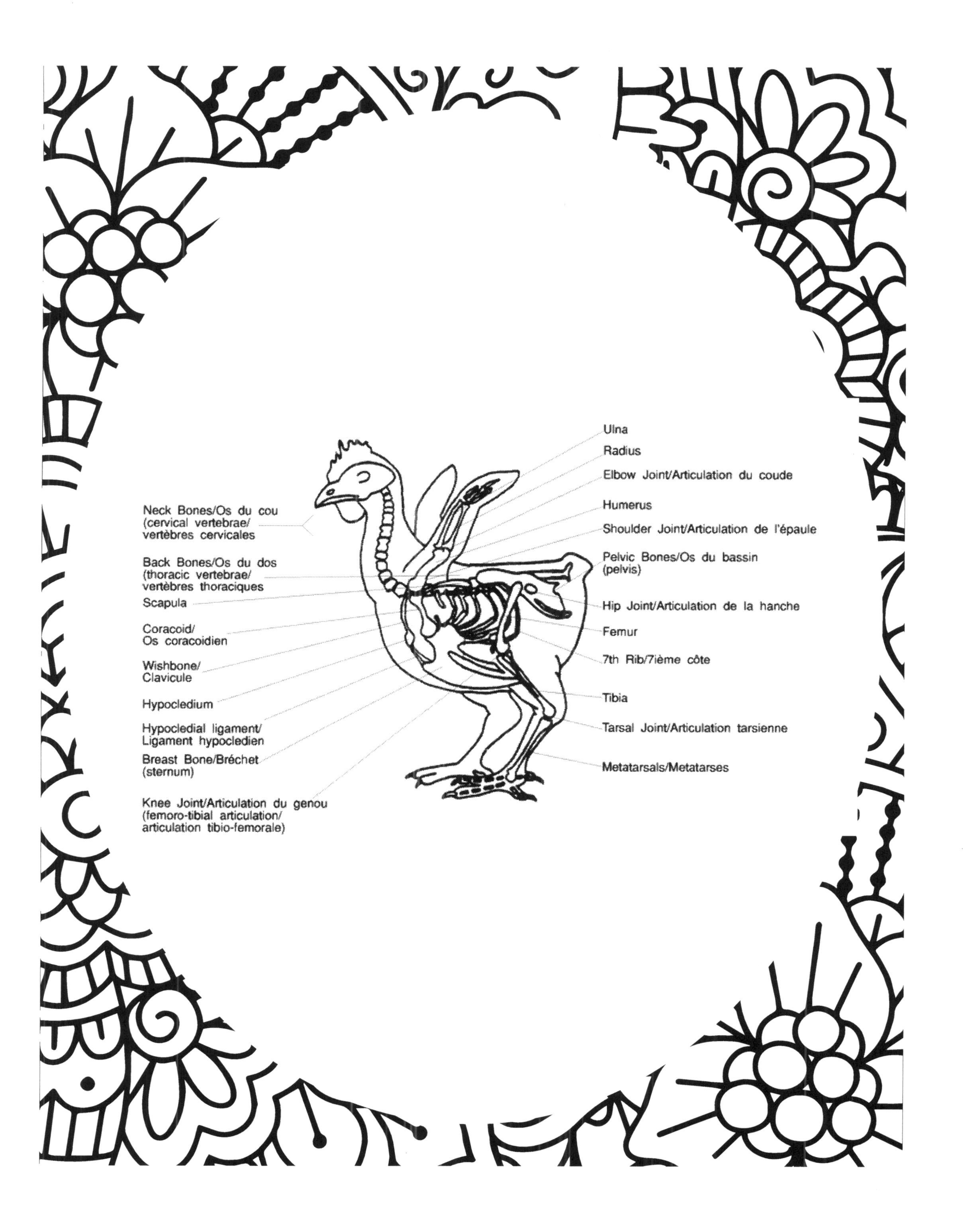
Ulna
Radius
Elbow Joint/Articulation du coude
Humerus
Shoulder Joint/Articulation de l'épaule
Pelvic Bones/Os du bassin
(pelvis)
Hip Joint/Articulation de la hanche
Femur
7th Rib/7ième côte
Tibia
Tarsal Joint/Articulation tarsienne
Metatarsals/Metatarses
Neck Bones/Os du cou
(cervical vertebrae/
vertèbres cervicales
Back Bones/Os du dos
(thoracic vertebrae/
vertèbres thoraciques
Scapula
Coracoid/
Os coracoidien
Wishbone/
Clavicule
Hypocledium
Hypocledial ligament/
Ligament hypocledien
Breast Bone/Bréchet
(sternum)
Knee Joint/Articulation du genou
(femoro-tibial articulation/
articulation tibio-femorale)

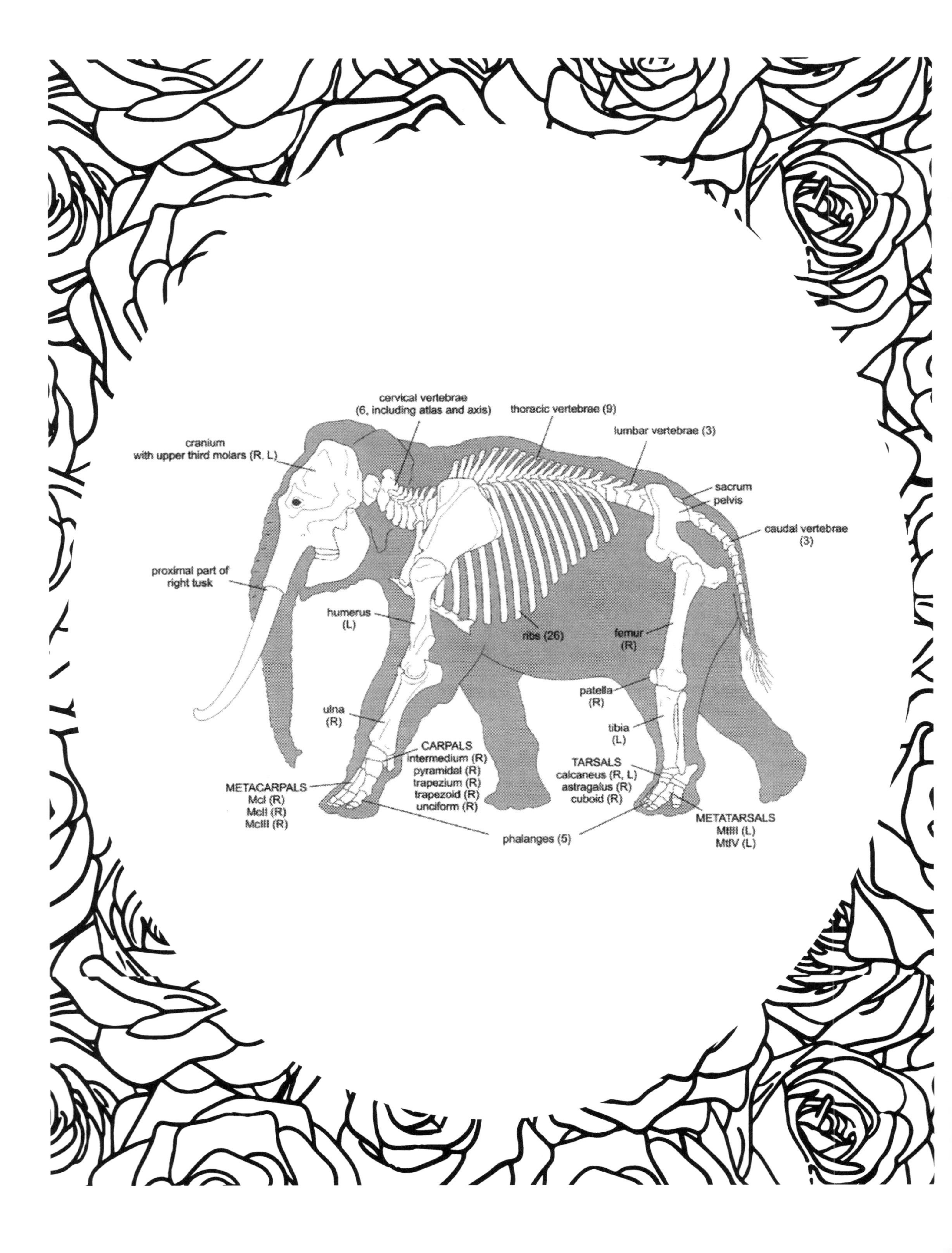
cervical vertebrae
(6, including atlas and axis)
thoracic vertebrae (9)
lumbar vertebrae (3)
cranium
with upper third molars (R, L)
sacrum
pelvis
caudal vertebrae
(3)
proximal part of
right tusk
humerus
(L)
ribs (26)
femur
(R)
patella
(R)
ulna
(R)
tibia
(L)
CARPALS
intermedium (R)
pyramidal (R)
trapezium (R)
trapezoid (R)
unciform (R)
TARSALS
calcaneus (R, L)
astragalus (R)
cuboid (R)
METACARPALS
McI (R)
McII (R)
McIII (R)
METATARSALS
MtIII (L)
MtIV (L)
phalanges (5)

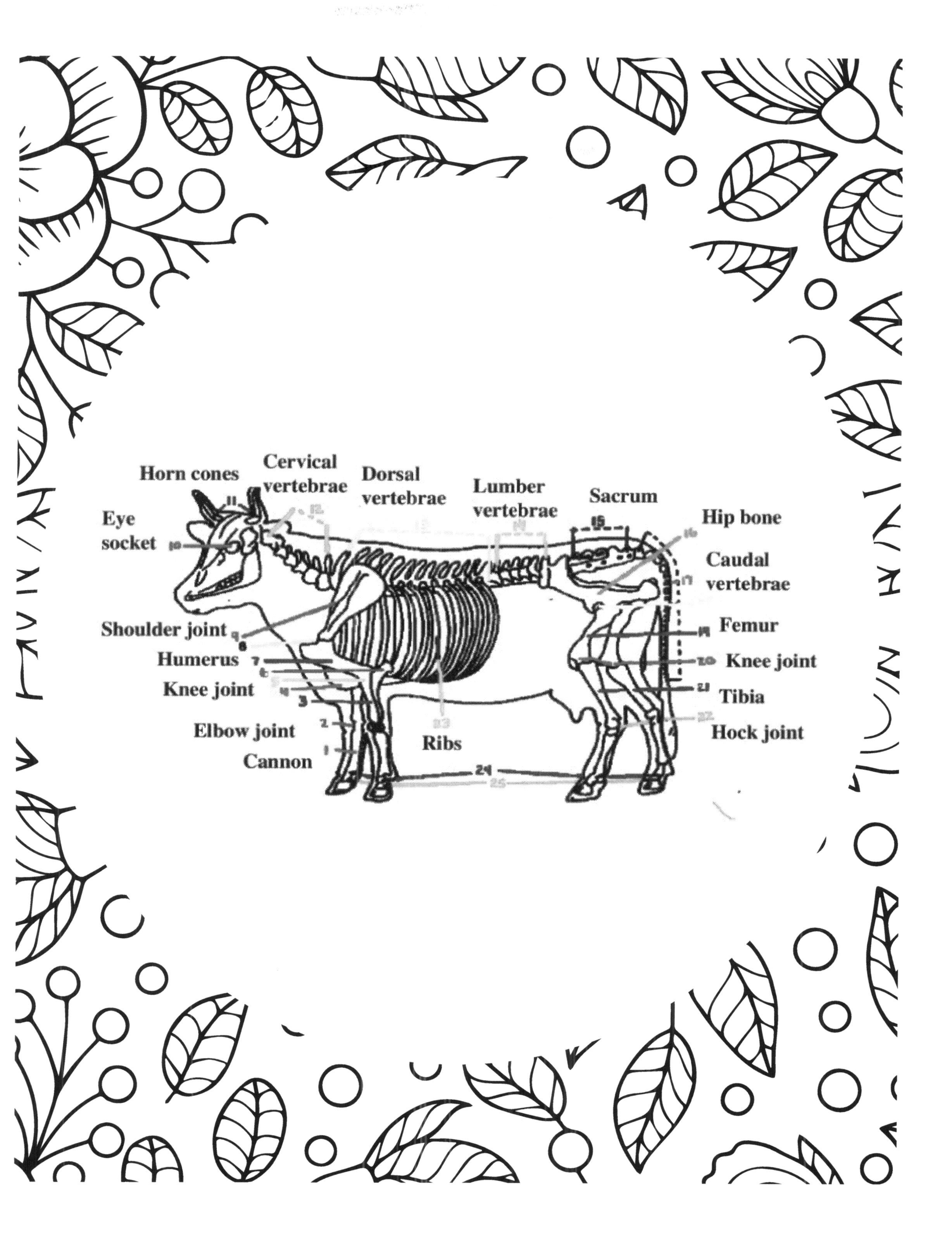

Horn cones
Cervical vertebrae
Dorsal vertebrae
Lumber vertebrae
Sacrum
Hip bone
Eye socket
Caudal vertebrae
Shoulder joint
Femur
Humerus
Knee joint
Knee joint
Tibia
Elbow joint
Hock joint
Ribs
Cannon

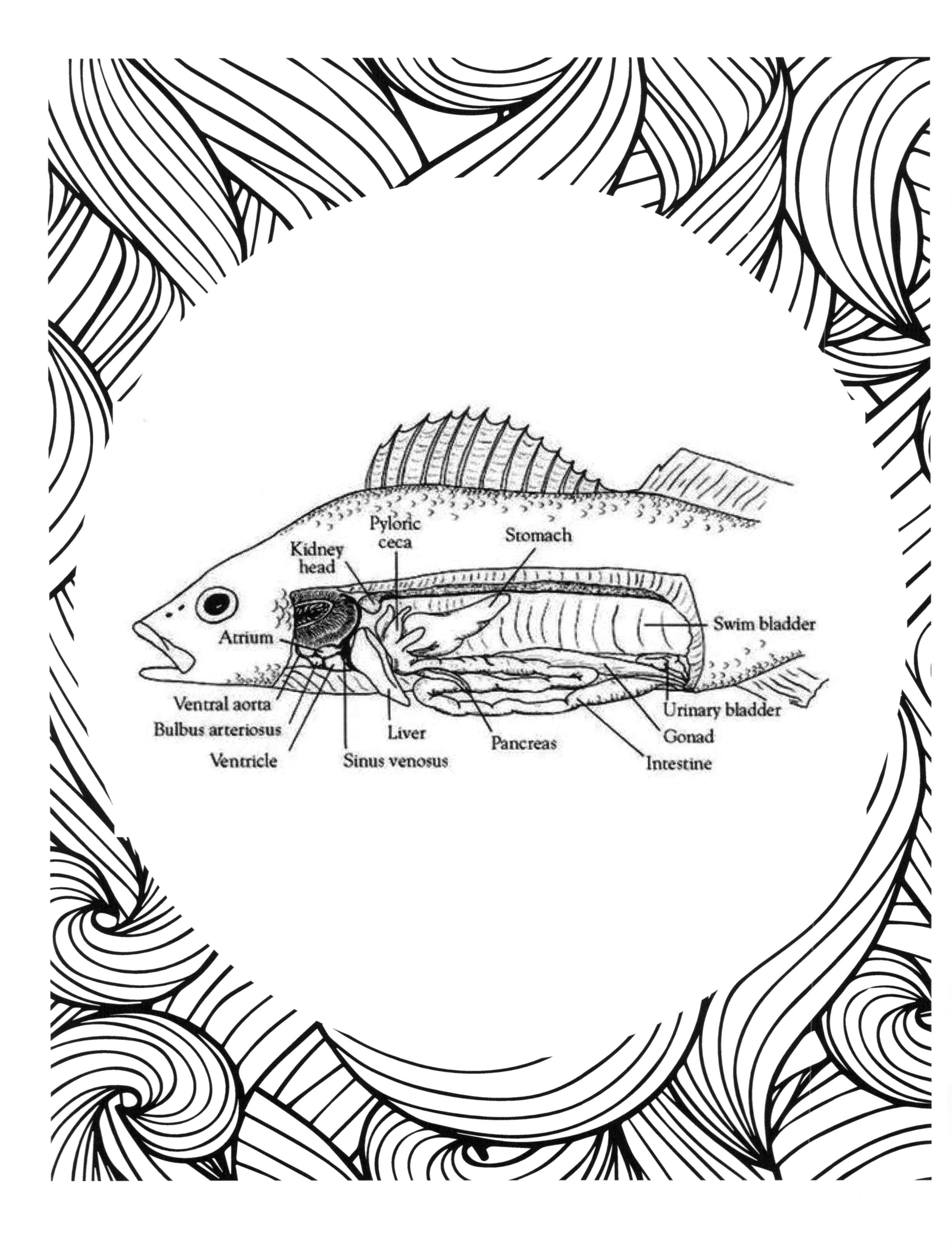
Pyloric ceca
Stomach
Kidney head
Swim bladder
Atrium
Ventral aorta
Urinary bladder
Bulbus arteriosus
Liver
Gonad
Pancreas
Ventricle
Sinus venosus
Intestine

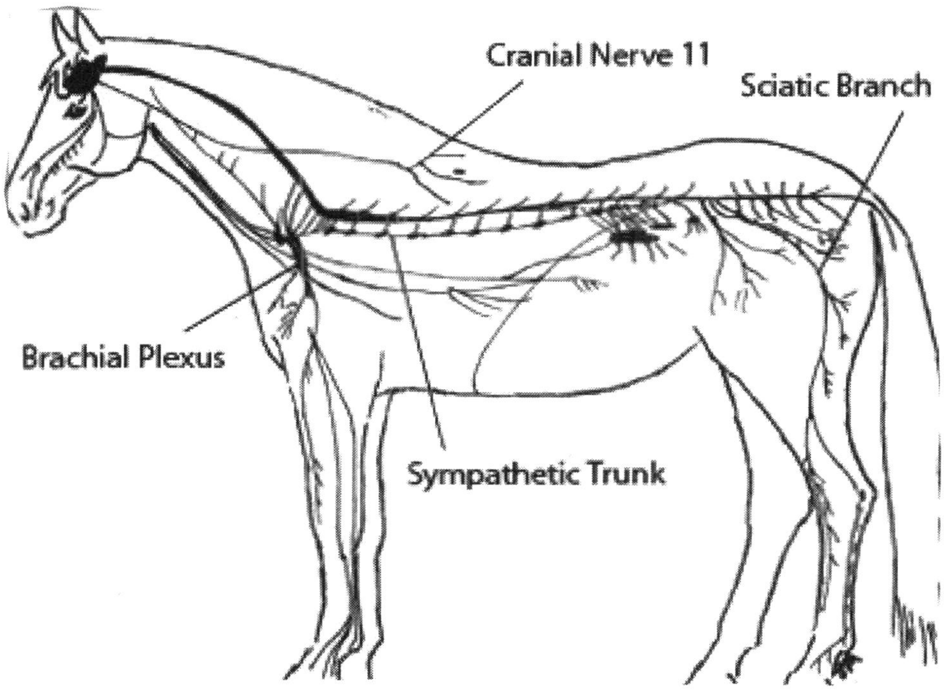

Cranial Nerve 11

Sciatic Branch

Brachial Plexus

Sympathetic Trunk

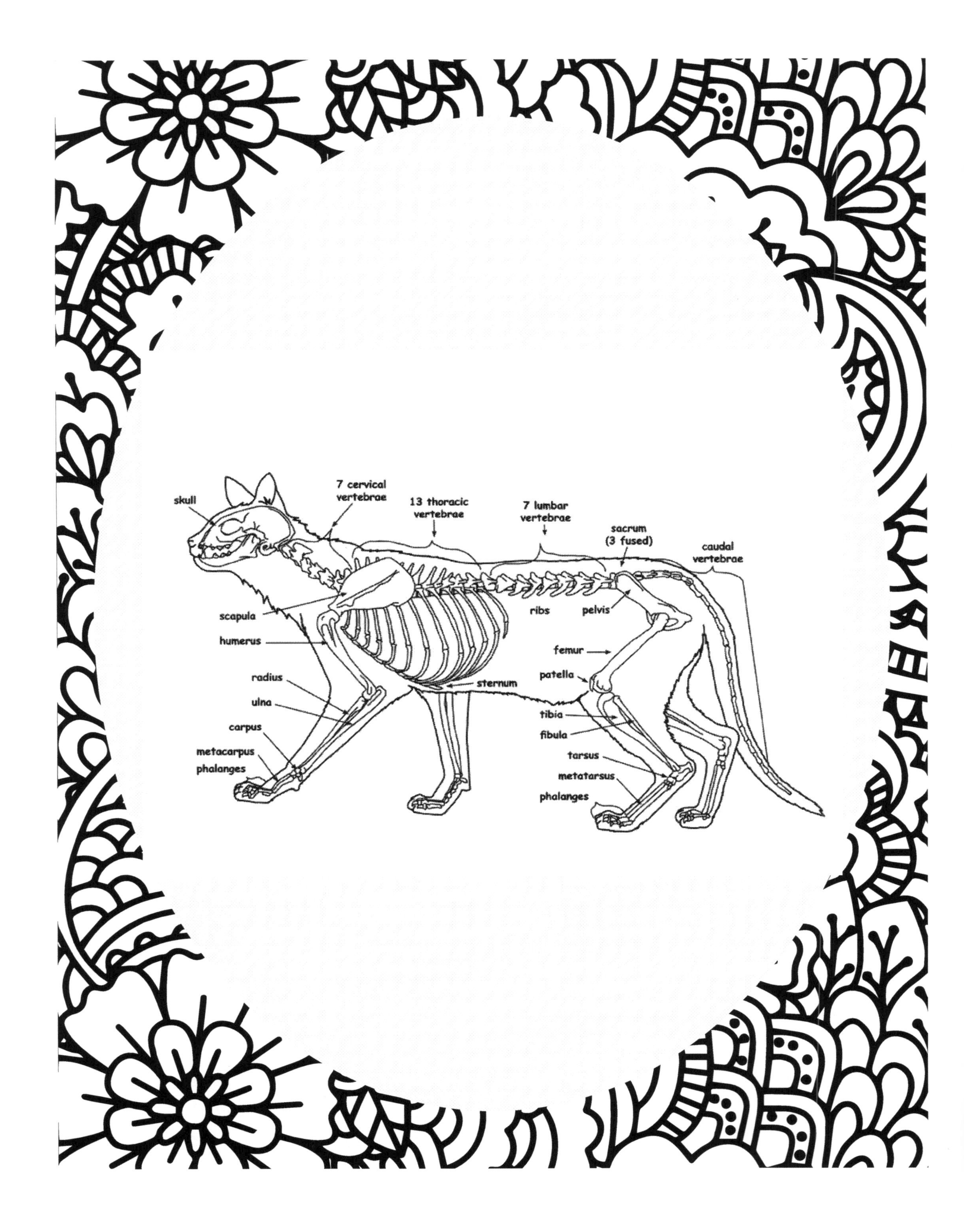

skull
7 cervical vertebrae
13 thoracic vertebrae
7 lumbar vertebrae
sacrum (3 fused)
caudal vertebrae
scapula
ribs
pelvis
humerus
femur
radius
patella
sternum
ulna
tibia
carpus
fibula
metacarpus
tarsus
phalanges
metatarsus
phalanges

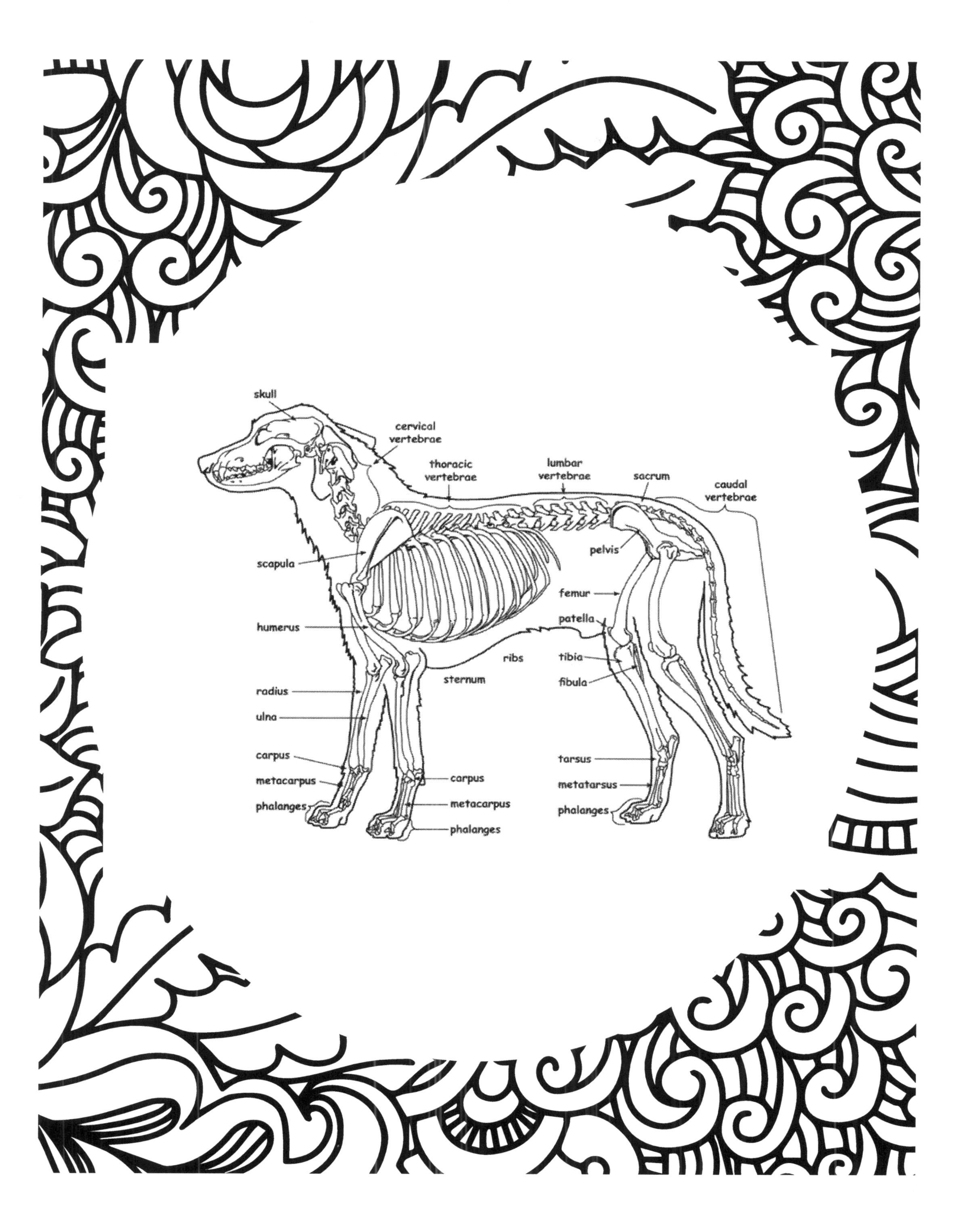
skull
cervical vertebrae
thoracic vertebrae
lumbar vertebrae
sacrum
caudal vertebrae
pelvis
scapula
femur
humerus
patella
ribs
tibia
sternum
fibula
radius
ulna
carpus
tarsus
carpus
metacarpus
metatarsus
metacarpus
phalanges
phalanges
phalanges

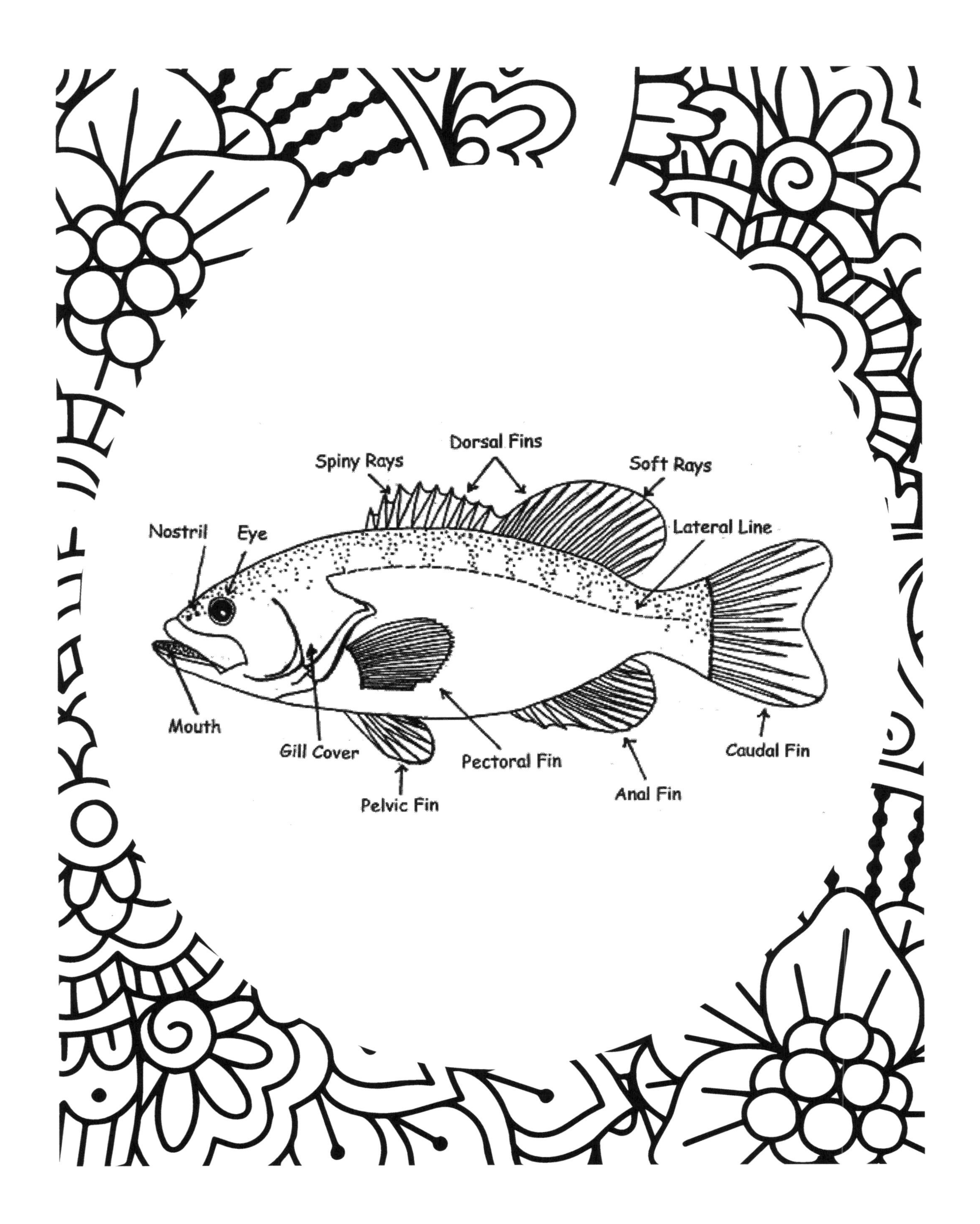
Dorsal Fins
Spiny Rays
Soft Rays
Nostril
Eye
Lateral Line
Mouth
Gill Cover
Pectoral Fin
Caudal Fin
Pelvic Fin
Anal Fin

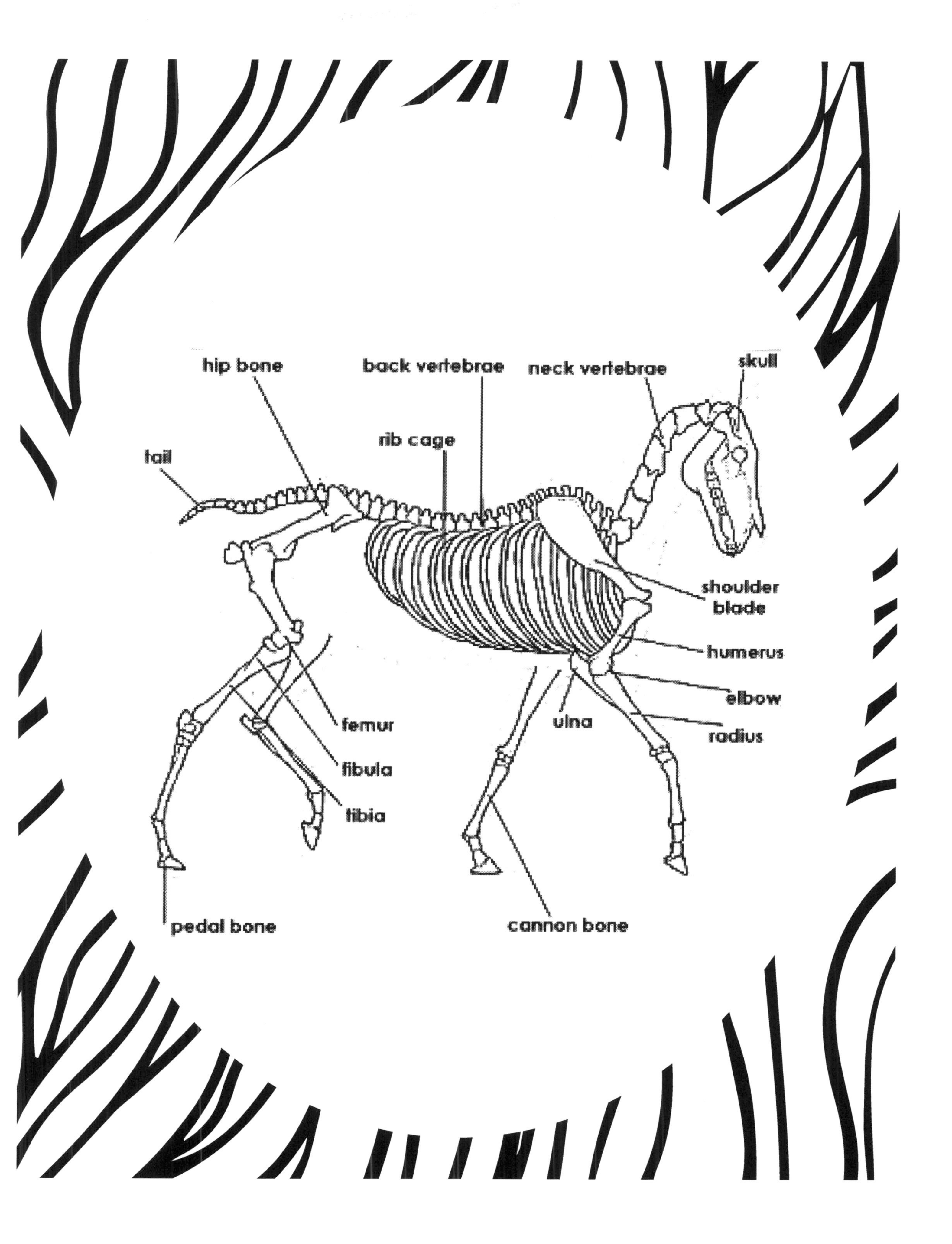
hip bone
back vertebrae
neck vertebrae
skull
rib cage
tail
shoulder
blade
humerus
elbow
femur
ulna
radius
fibula
tibia
pedal bone
cannon bone

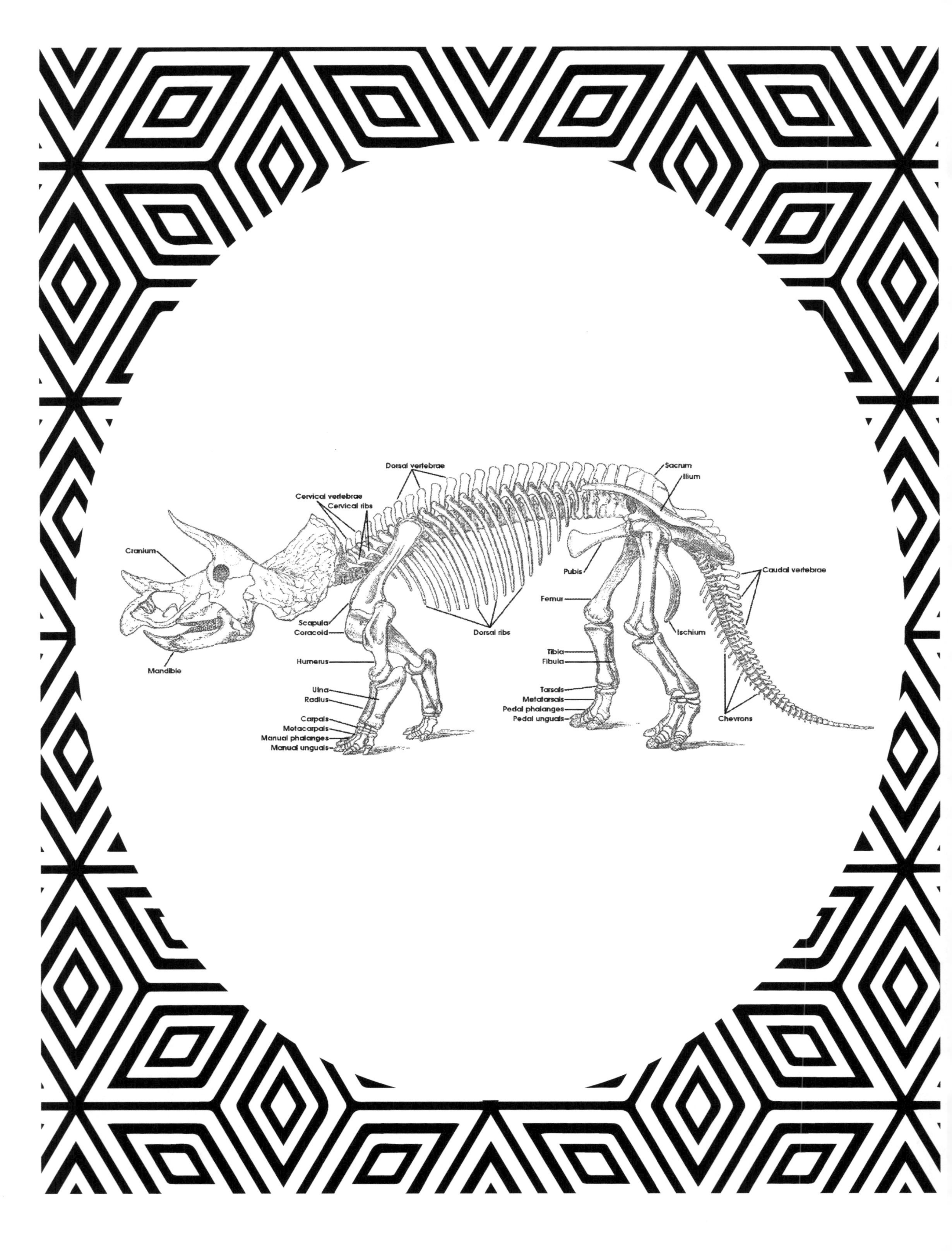

Dorsal vertebrae
Sacrum
Ilium
Cervical vertebrae
Cervical ribs
Cranium
Pubis
Caudal vertebrae
Femur
Scapula
Coracoid
Dorsal ribs
Ischium
Mandible
Tibia
Fibula
Humerus
Ulna
Radius
Tarsals
Metatarsals
Pedal phalanges
Pedal unguals
Chevrons
Carpals
Metacarpals
Manual phalanges
Manual unguals

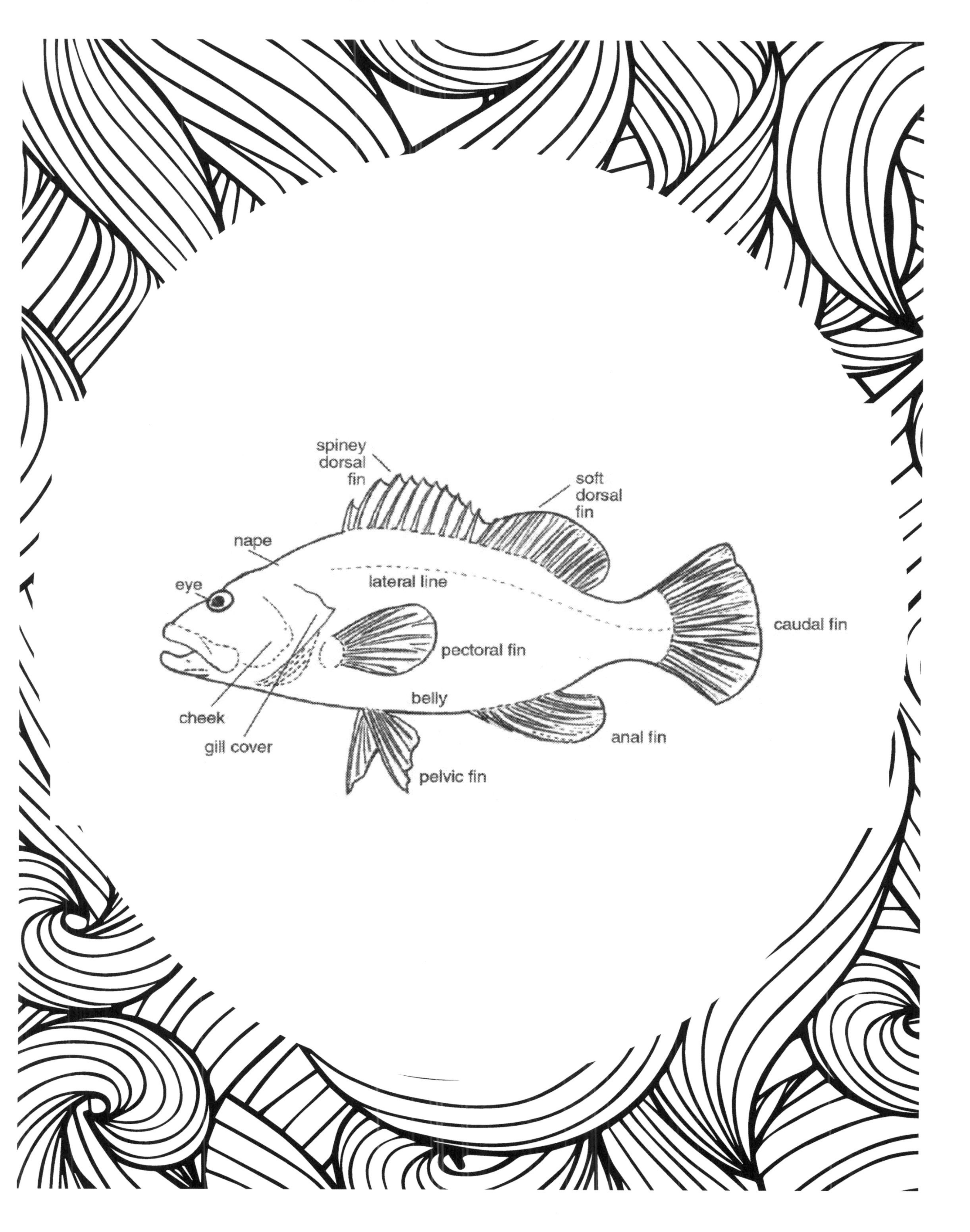
spiney
dorsal
fin
soft
dorsal
fin
nape
eye
lateral line
caudal fin
pectoral fin
belly
cheek
gill cover
anal fin
pelvic fin

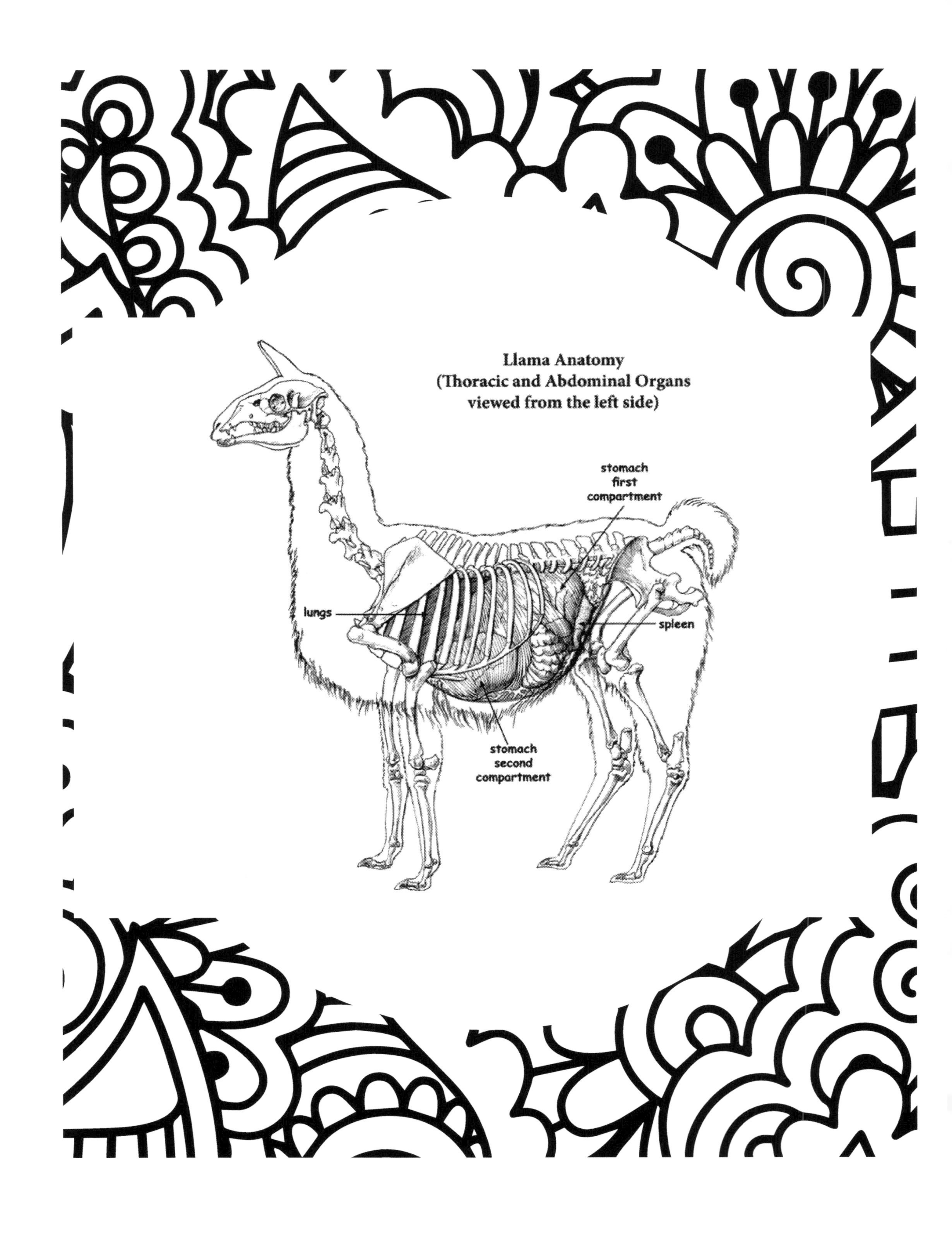
Llama Anatomy
(Thoracic and Abdominal Organs
viewed from the left side)
stomach
first
compartment
lungs
spleen
stomach
second
compartment

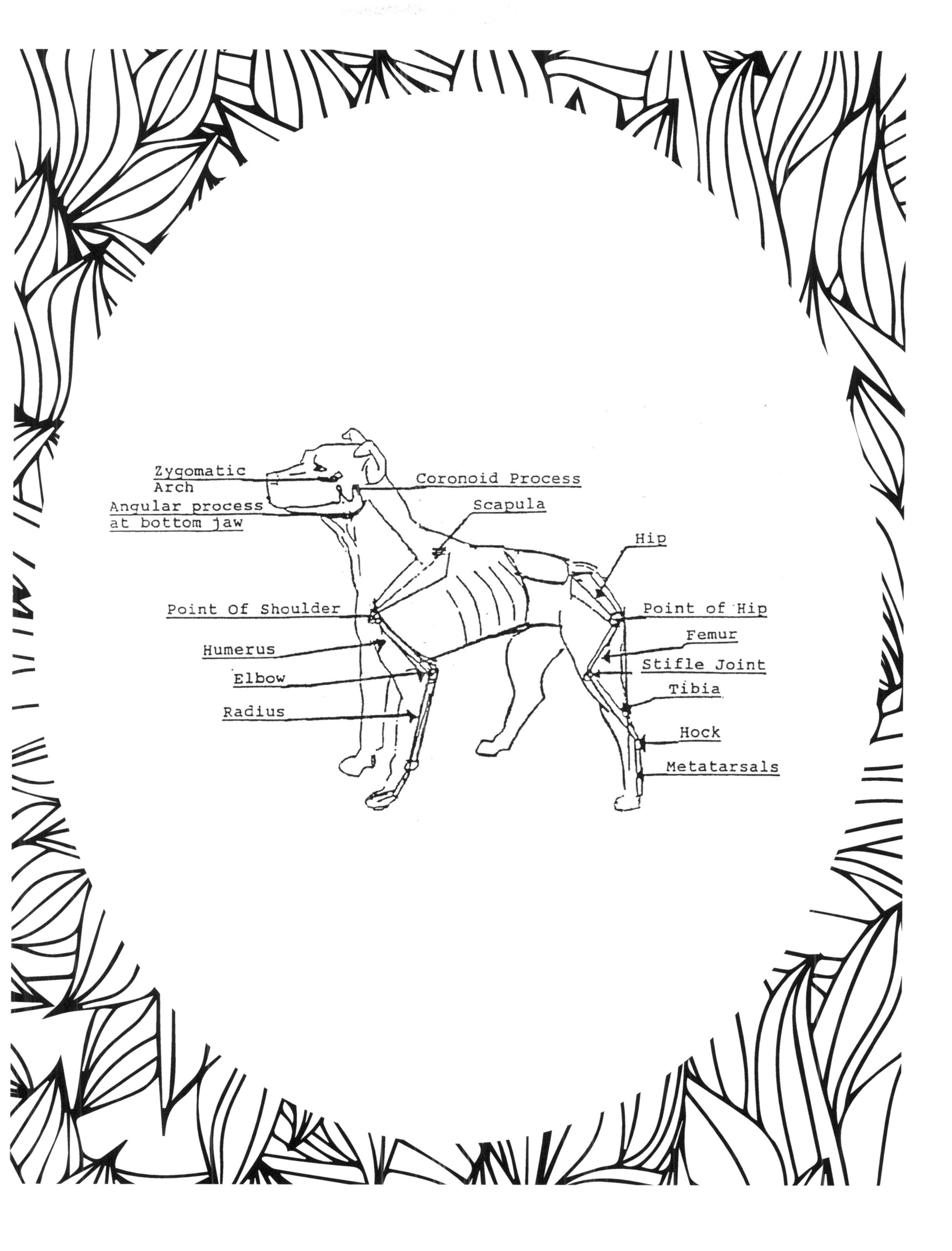
Zygomatic
Arch
Angular process
at bottom jaw
Coronoid Process
Scapula
Hip
Point Of Shoulder
Point of Hip
Humerus
Femur
Stifle Joint
Elbow
Tibia
Radius
Hock
Metatarsals

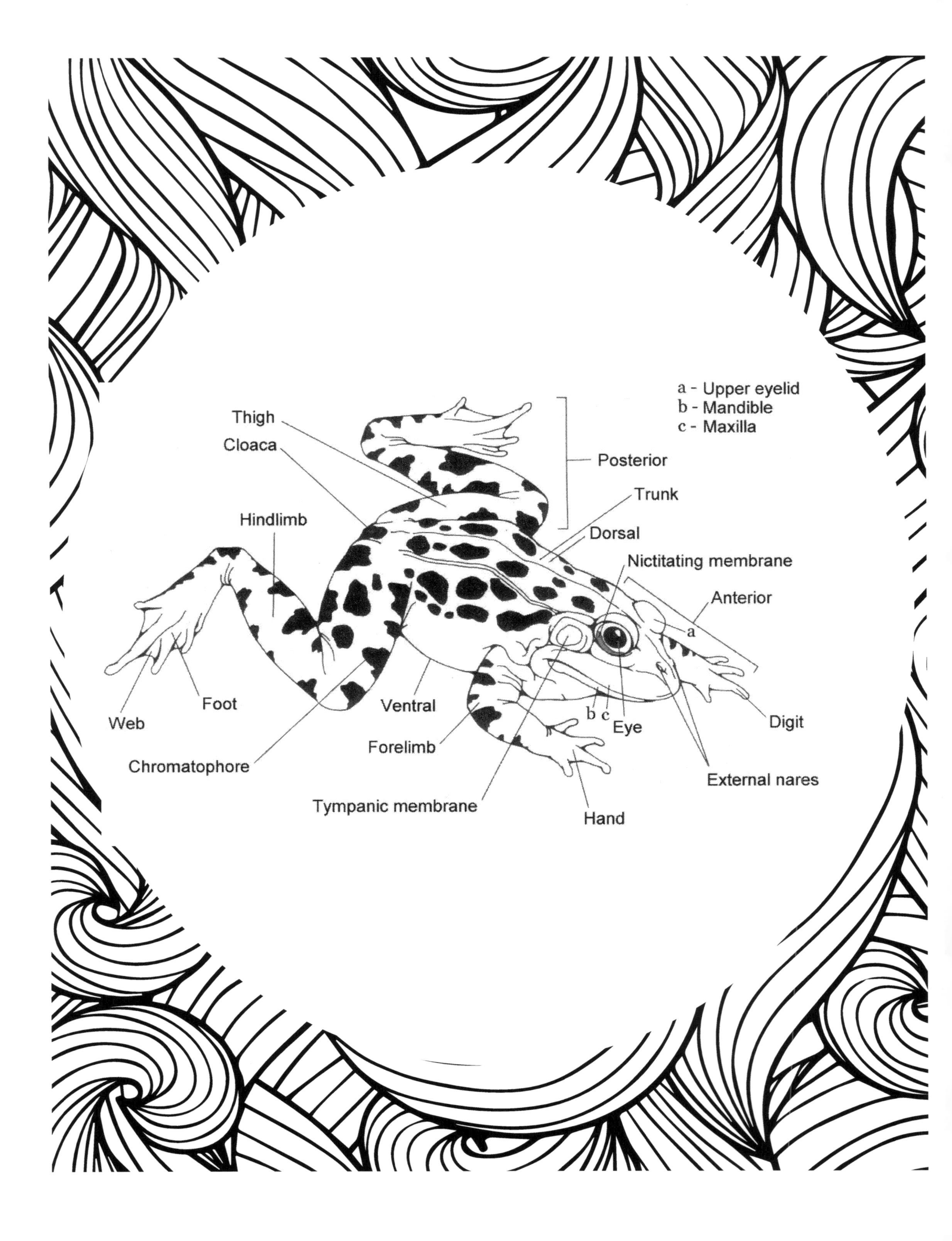
a - Upper eyelid
b - Mandible
c - Maxilla
Thigh
Cloaca
Posterior
Trunk
Hindlimb
Dorsal
Nictitating membrane
Anterior
a
Web
Foot
Ventral
b c
Eye
Digit
Forelimb
Chromatophore
External nares
Tympanic membrane
Hand

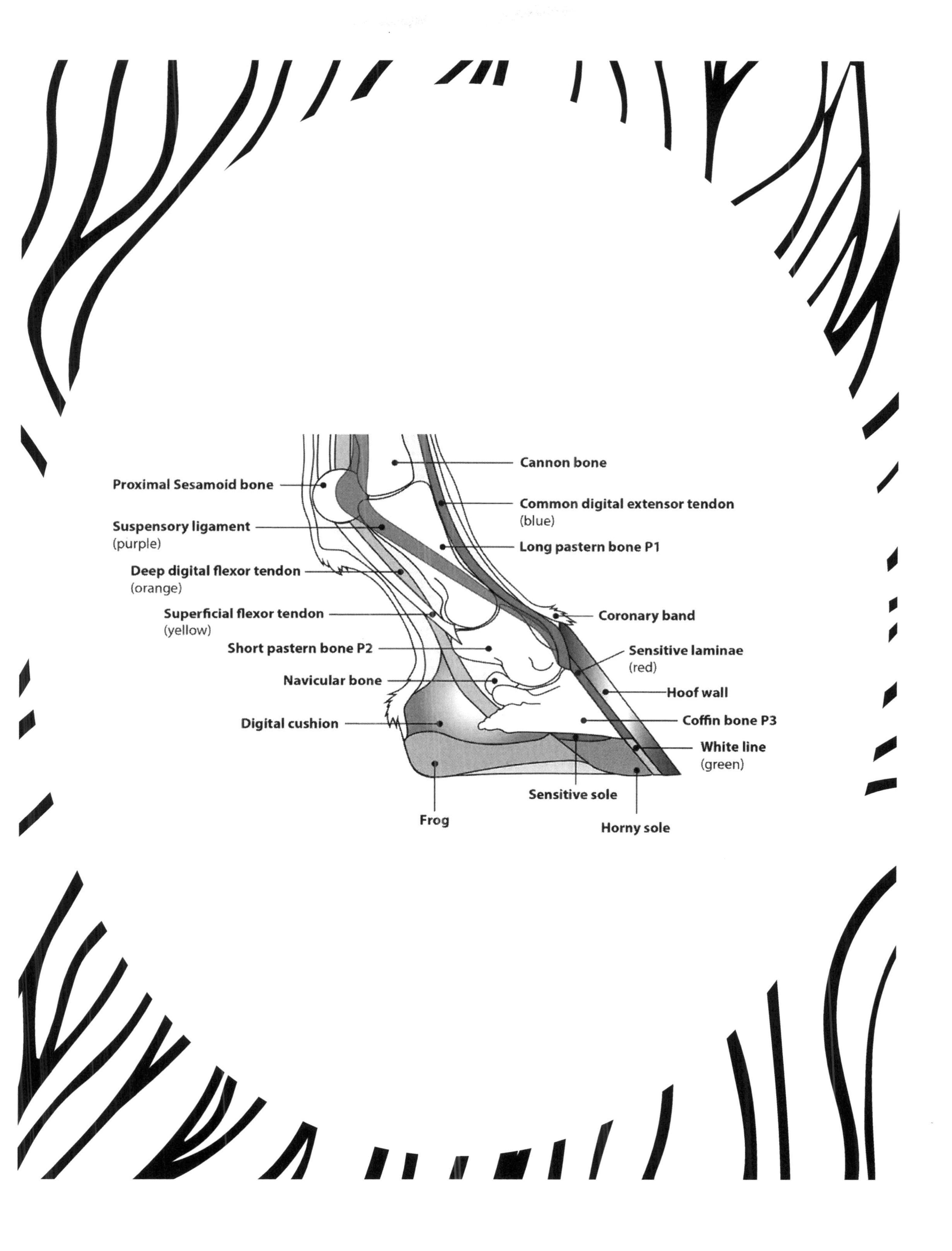
Cannon bone
Proximal Sesamoid bone
Common digital extensor tendon
(blue)
Suspensory ligament
(purple)
Long pastern bone P1
Deep digital flexor tendon
(orange)
Superficial flexor tendon
(yellow)
Coronary band
Short pastern bone P2
Sensitive laminae
(red)
Navicular bone
Hoof wall
Digital cushion
Coffin bone P3
White line
(green)
Sensitive sole
Frog
Horny sole

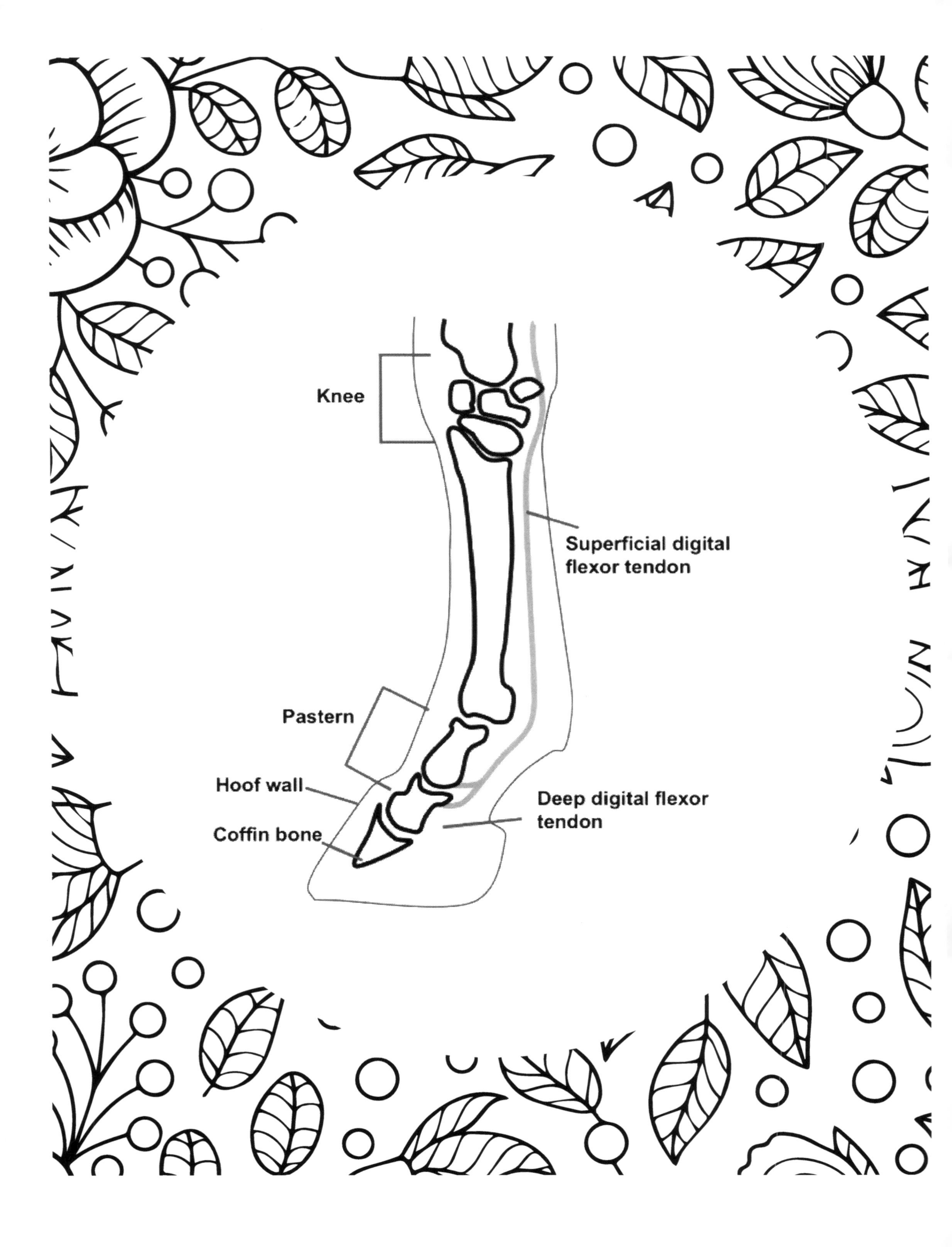
Knee
Superficial digital flexor tendon
Pastern
Hoof wall
Deep digital flexor tendon
Coffin bone

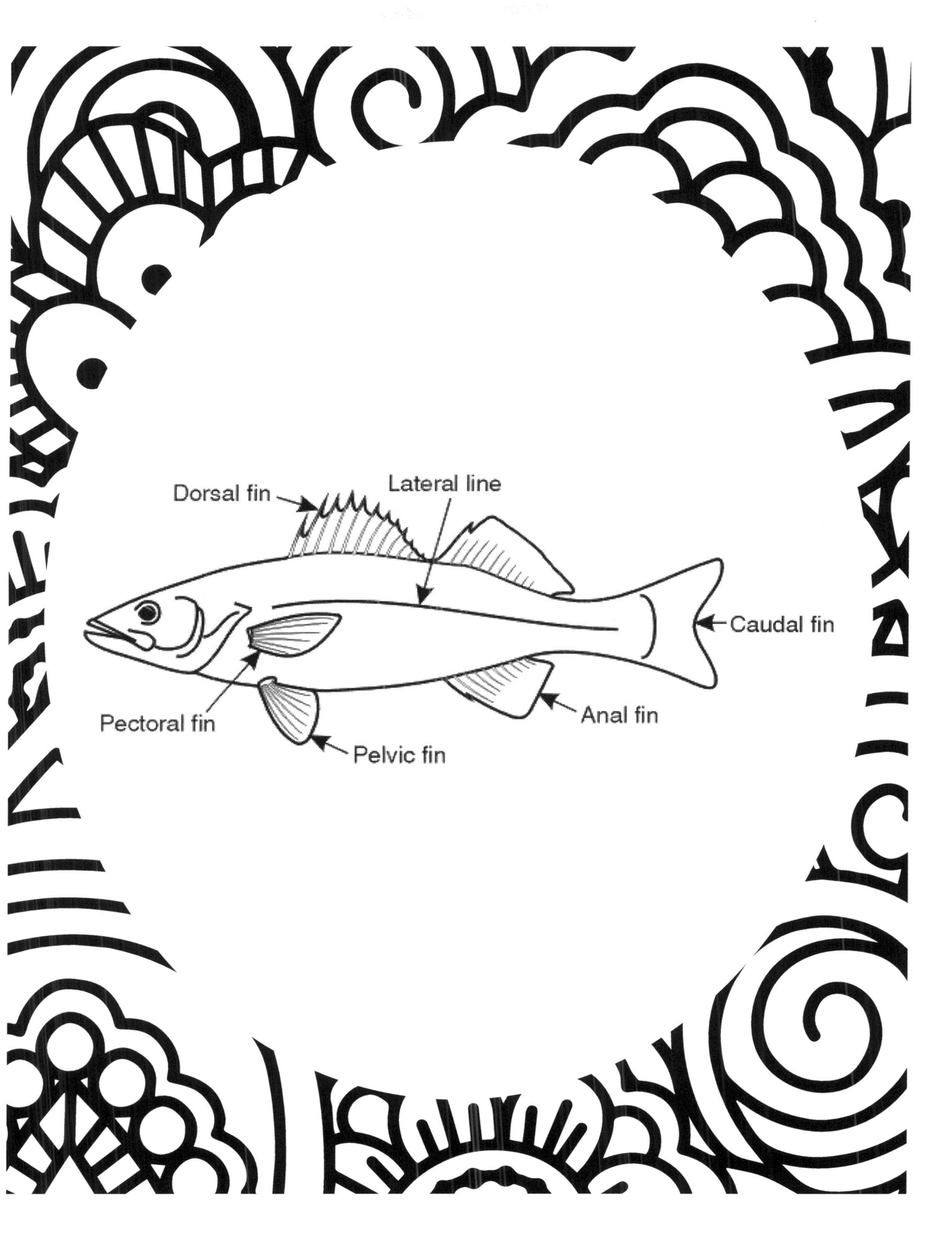
Dorsal fin
Lateral line
Caudal fin
Pectoral fin
Anal fin
Pelvic fin

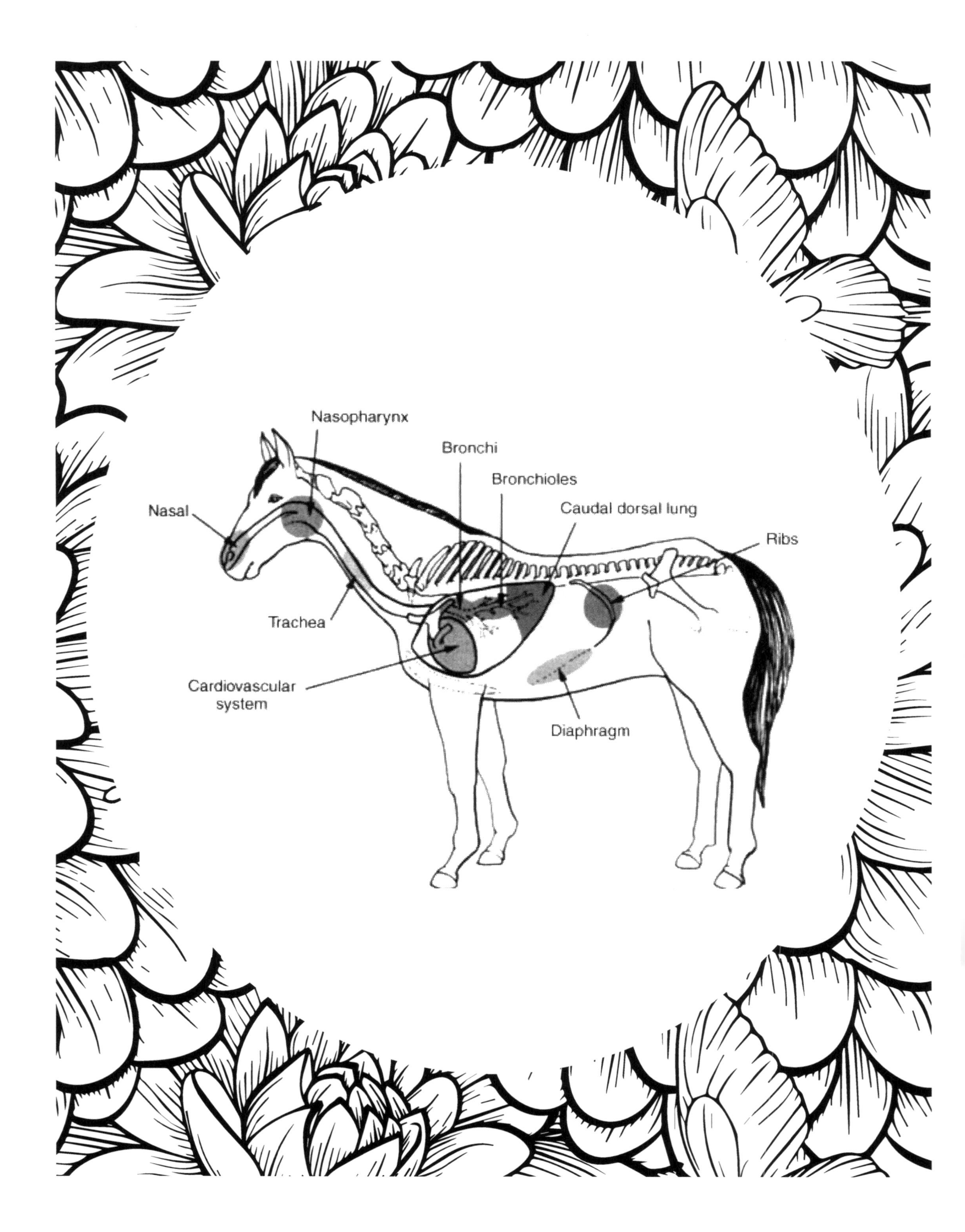
Nasopharynx
Bronchi
Bronchioles
Caudal dorsal lung
Nasal
Ribs
Trachea
Cardiovascular
system
Diaphragm

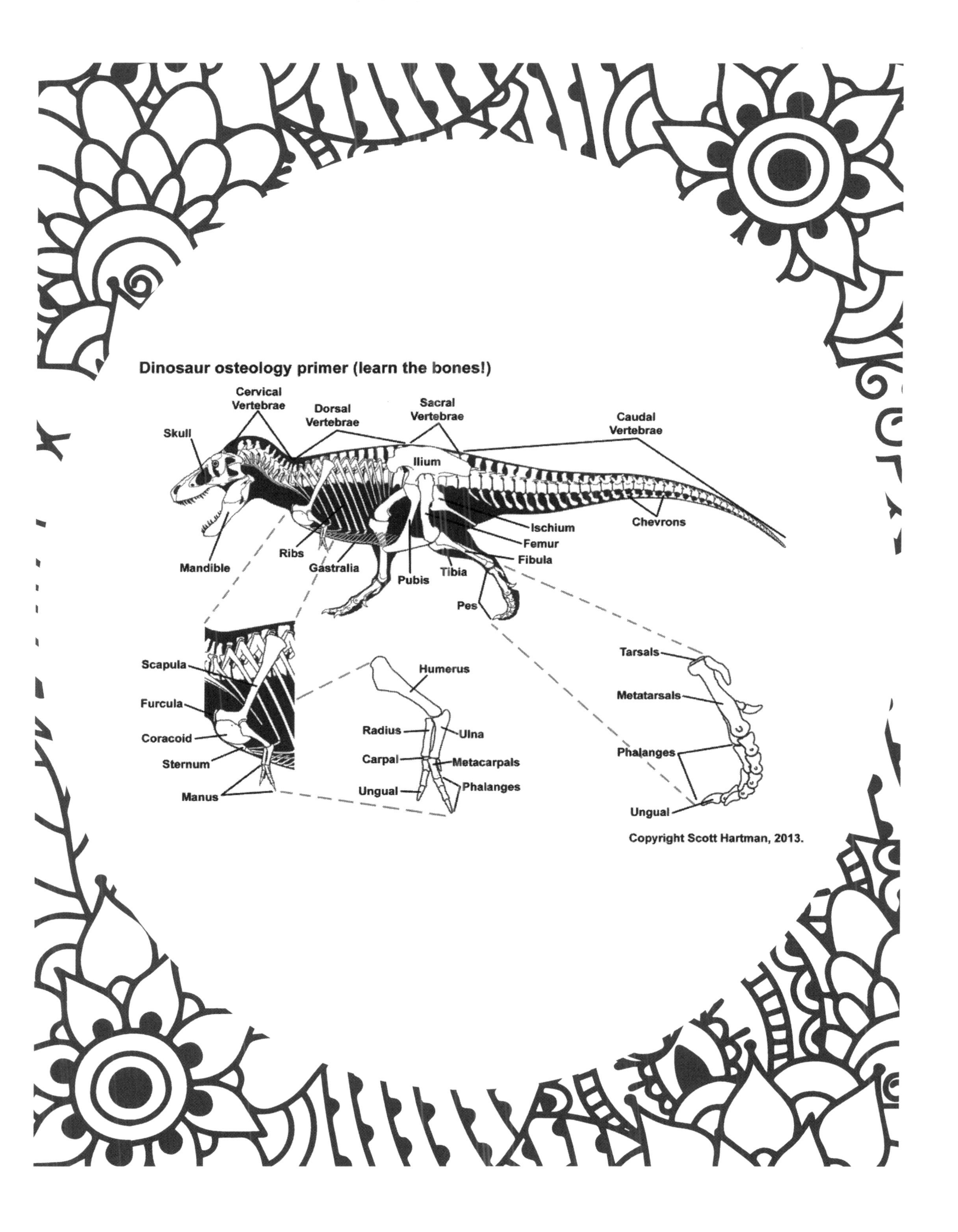
Dinosaur osteology primer (learn the bones!)
Cervical Vertebrae
Dorsal Vertebrae
Sacral Vertebrae
Caudal Vertebrae
Skull
Ilium
Chevrons
Ischium
Femur
Fibula
Mandible
Ribs
Gastralia
Pubis
Tibia
Pes
Scapula
Furcula
Coracoid
Sternum
Manus
Humerus
Radius
Ulna
Carpal
Metacarpals
Ungual
Phalanges
Tarsals
Metatarsals
Phalanges
Ungual
Copyright Scott Hartman, 2013.

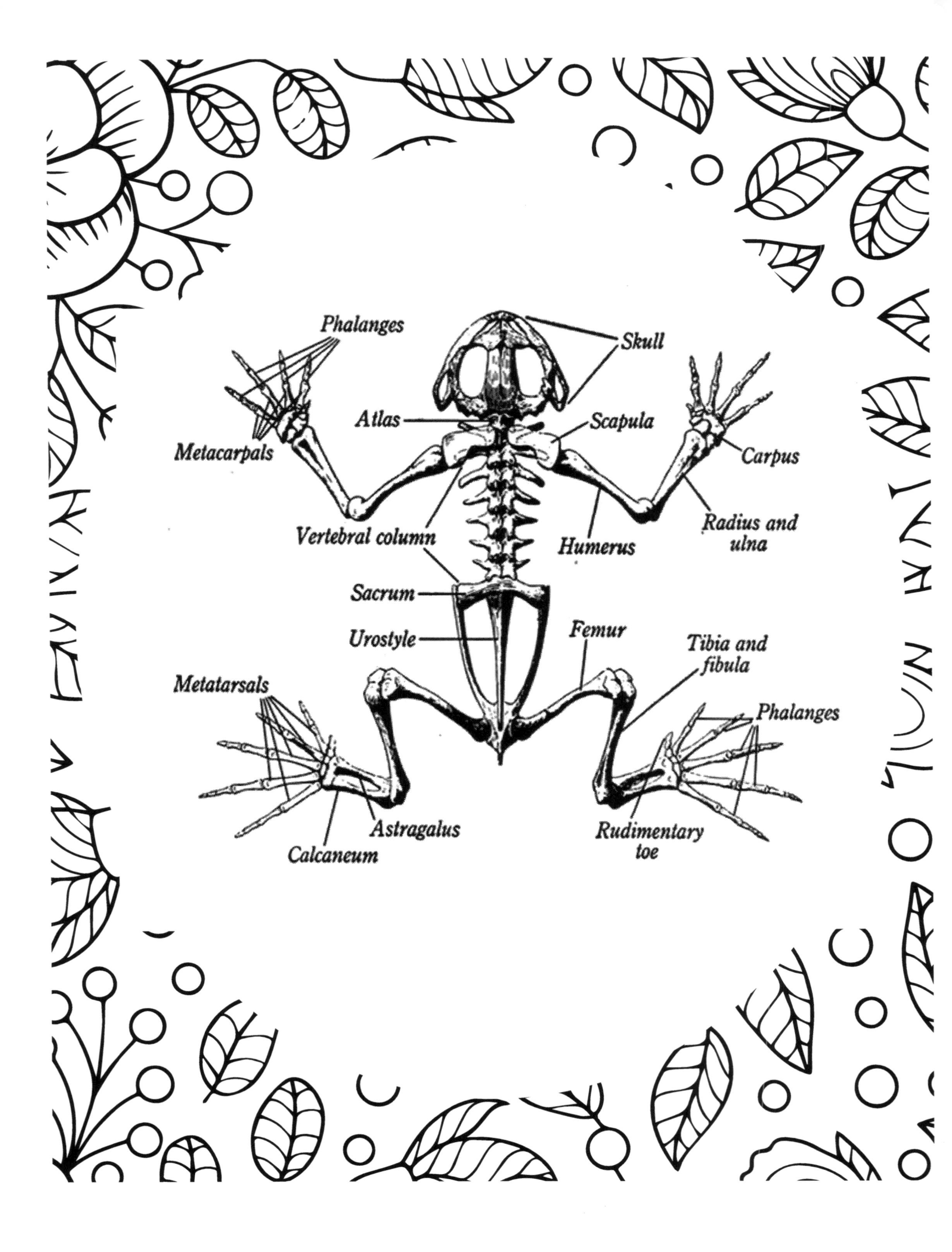
Phalanges
Skull
Atlas
Scapula
Metacarpals
Carpus
Vertebral column
Humerus
Radius and ulna
Sacrum
Urostyle
Femur
Tibia and fibula
Metatarsals
Phalanges
Astragalus
Calcaneum
Rudimentary toe

Printed in Great Britain
by Amazon

63645482R00029